Supporting

Breast feeding

Past the First Six Months and Beyond

of related interest

Supporting Queer Birth
A Book for Birth Professionals and Parents
AJ Silver
ISBN 978 1 83997 045 0
eISBN 978 1 83997 046 7

Breastfeeding Twins and Triplets
A Guide for Professionals and Parents
Kathryn Stagg
ISBN 978 1 83997 049 8
eISBN 978 1 83997 050 4

Supporting Autistic Women through Pregnancy and Childbirth
Hayley Morgan, Emma Durman and Dr Alys Einion-Waller
ISBN 978 1 83997 105 1
eISBN 978 1 83997 106 8

Weaving the Cradle
Facilitating Groups to Promote Attunement and Bonding between Parents, Their Babies and Toddlers
Edited by Monika Celebi
Foreword by Jane Barlow
ISBN 978 1 84819 311 6
eISBN 978 0 85701 264 7

Supporting Breastfeeding Past the First Six Months and Beyond

A Guide for Professionals and Parents

Emma Pickett

Illustrated by JoJo Ford

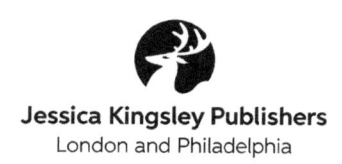

Jessica Kingsley Publishers
London and Philadelphia

First published in Great Britain in 2022 by Jessica Kingsley Publishers
An imprint of Hodder & Stoughton Ltd
An Hachette UK Company

1

Copyright © Emma Pickett 2022

The right of Emma Pickett to be identified as the Author of the Work has been asserted by her in accordance with the Copyright, Designs and Patents Act 1988.

All rights reserved. No part of this publication may be reproduced, stored in a retrieval system, or transmitted, in any form or by any means without the prior written permission of the publisher, nor be otherwise circulated in any form of binding or cover other than that in which it is published and without a similar condition being imposed on the subsequent purchaser.

A CIP catalogue record for this title is available from the
British Library and the Library of Congress

ISBN 978 1 78775 989 3
eISBN 978 1 78775 990 9

Printed and bound in Great Britain by CPI Group

Jessica Kingsley Publishers' policy is to use papers that are natural, renewable and recyclable products and made from wood grown in sustainable forests. The logging and manufacturing processes are expected to conform to the environmental regulations of the country of origin.

Jessica Kingsley Publishers
Carmelite House
50 Victoria Embankment
London EC4Y 0DZ

www.jkp.com

Breastfeeding Lu brought me home to my body. For most of my life I've tried to make my body fit this ideal that floated around in my mind. Carrying and birthing my baby made me realize how astonishing my body is. And breastfeeding him has helped me accept, love and like my body. I now view my body with kindness, patience and awe. Being able to meet my nursing goals did that, and I was able to meet them with the love and support of others, and for this I am forever grateful. Every parent deserves that – the chance to feed their baby how they choose, to be listened to, to be supported, to be given the time, to be seen. Each baby deserves the chance to breastfeed. Every time I breastfeed my son I feel like I'm in my truest home and I hope that it helps him to feel his body is his truest home too.

~ (Michelle)

For those who advocate for parents to be able to breastfeed for as long as they want to.

Contents

Acknowledgements 9

Notes on the Text 10

1. Introduction 11

2. Let's Celebrate Getting to Six Months and the Value in Continuing 29

3. Conversations with Others and the Role of the Partner 48

4. Solid Food Alongside Breastfeeding 76

5. Breastfeeding and Sleep 93

6. Returning to Work 110

7. Nursing Manners and Communicating Limits 131

8. Common Problems and Challenges 146

9. Getting Pregnant Again 176

10. Ending Breastfeeding 199

11. Family Stories 232

References 267

Further Resources 278

Suject Index 280

Author Index 285

Acknowledgements

This book would not have been possible without the contributions of all the parents who shared their stories with me. Thank you to Aisling, Alice, Alison, Amy, Ashley, BJ, Becky, Bertille, Camila, Camilla, Caprice, Carly, Catherine, Daisy, Elizabeth, Emily, Emma, Evelyn, Fi, Freya, Hannah, Jes, Kathryn, Kim, Kimberley, Lauren, Lucy, Lucy, Manni, Maria, Meera, Meg, Michelle, Milda, Mira, Miriam, Naomi, Natalie, Natasha, Nicola, Rachael, Rachel, Rhian, Ruth, Sandra, Sarah, Saskia, Sharon, Sophie, Tamzin, Toby, Vanisha and Zoe.

Thank you to the parents whom I have supported and who have inspired me, especially members of the Wednesday and Thursday clubs.

Thank you also to Camila Palma, Richa Sharma, Lucy Upton, Paula Hallam, Stacey Zimmels, Marina Ferrari, Lyndsey Hookway, Ali Thomas and Sally Dowling for your valuable contributions. Thank you, Vicky Thomas, for your thoughts and your beautiful poem.

JoJo Ford, I love your illustrations and it is always a pleasure to work with you. Thank you to Jessica Kingsley Publishers and especially Maddy Budd. Thank you to Gabrielle Chambers for your help with editing.

Notes on the Text

This book is written from the perspective of a parent who breastfed and raised children in the UK and supports UK parents as a professional. The interviews with other families are largely UK-focused and the observations mainly explore the experiences of those living in W.E.I.R.D. countries (Western, Educated, Industrialized, Rich and Democratic). These countries may possess only a minority of the world's population but are often struggling with supporting families in reaching their breastfeeding goals and feeding beyond six months. Conversely, five countries in the world have a 90% breastfeeding rate from 6 to 23 months: Nepal, Rwanda, Ethiopia, Burundi and Guinea (Rollins *et al.* 2016). All quotes given by parents and professionals were shared with the author either via interview or in written form in 2020 and 2021 and consent was given for publication. This includes a conversation with Sally Dowling and conversations with some parents who asked not to have their names shared.

    Lactation support is about centring the families we support and helping them on their personal journeys at a time when they may often feel isolated. Not all parents who feed their children beyond six months use the terms 'mothers' and 'breastfeeding'. I use the term 'breastfeeding' in this text, but when speaking to some parents 'nursing' or 'chestfeeding' may be more appropriate.

    This book's content is for informational purposes only and is not intended to serve as a substitute for the consultation, diagnosis and/or medical treatment of a qualified physician or healthcare provider.

Chapter 1

Introduction

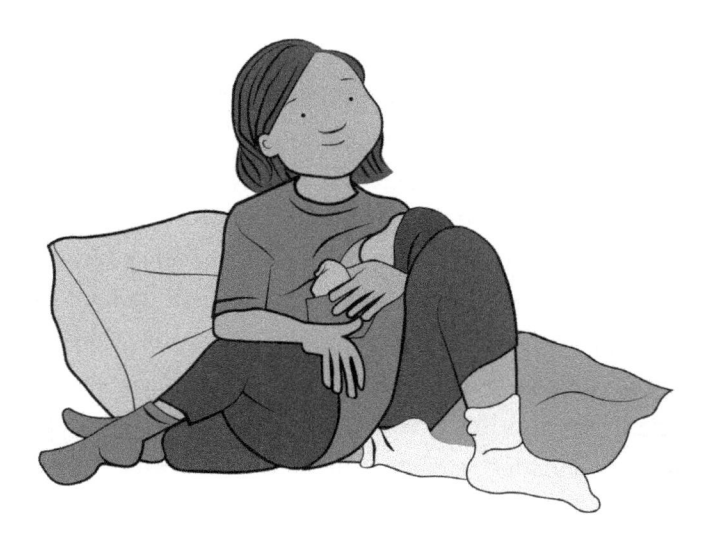

Families who breastfeed beyond six months are not all the same. There is no one unifying feature, other than the fact a small person is taking milk from a big person and the small person has been alive for at least half a year. They don't all think the same, not even about the fact that they are still breastfeeding. They may have had very few difficulties, cruised along successfully and needed minimal health professional input, certainly not about the breastfeeding itself. They may not need very much support from us at all. It may have been a straightforward day-to-day journey. Breastfeeding an older child is ordinary. It's been the default position for hundreds of thousands of years. It's humans on their 'factory settings'.

For others, the experience may have been stressful and challenging. They may have felt trapped, exhausted but still persevered. Breastfeeding an older child is not universally sitting on blankets in sunny meadows and thanking each day. In many cases, dealing with the assumptions and attitudes of others will have been one of the more stressful components.

Breastfeeding families don't have the same goals and daily experiences, and their nursling may come to the breast for very different reasons. For some, breastfeeding is one aspect of parenting that sits alongside dozens of other tools. For other families, breastfeeding is not an act but a relationship. It is central to their identity and at the heart of their parenting life.

Let's picture two different ten-month-old babies: One may breastfeed in the morning on waking and again around bedtime, before rolling over and falling asleep. For him, breastfeeding is a small part of a rich and varied diet, has very little to do with the process of falling asleep and is not the most important part of life. For another ten-month-old, the breast is the centre of their universe. They will wake to breastfeed having co-slept and breastfed throughout the night. They may easily wake every 90 minutes. They will request a breastfeed throughout the day, especially when feeling tired or upset. Solid food is part of their diet but the nutritional contribution of breastmilk is by far the majority. If you were to ask their parent how often they breastfed, the answer would probably be a hunch of the shoulders.

The second ten-month-old's parent comes to a clinic to meet with a health professional. What response will they receive? It may be anything from a 'Well done' to a 'Why are you still doing that?' When you read a description of that day of constant breastfeeding, what did you picture? Did you imagine a parent at their wit's end? Or did you imagine a happy household where breastfeeding was a positive parenting tool and adults were more than happy with the current situation? Did one of those ten-month-olds feel 'normal' and the other feel a concern? Where do those assumptions come from? Meg, a doctor in general practice in the UK: 'I find health professional attitudes reflect personal experience. Health professionals who have breastfed (or whose partners have) tend to value it more than those who haven't.'

That assumes the parent is even going to describe their daily life accurately once at the clinic:

> I just lied to them in the early days. I answered the questions the way I knew they should be answered as I didn't want to hear their poor advice nor have to justify myself and my choices to them.
>
> ~ *(Daisy, who breastfed her two children beyond babyhood)*

Of course, health professionals are often very supportive: they save breastfeeding relationships every day whether as lactation consultants, paediatricians, nurses, health visitors or midwives. But once breastfeeding continues past the first six months and beyond the first and second years, more health professionals seem to struggle with understanding how best to support families in their care. As Meg (the doctor quoted above) suggests, 'This is not with any ill intent, it is simply a lack of understanding of the value of breastfeeding.'

Our society likes to place people into boxes. *These* are the people who are new parents. *These* people are pregnant and breastfeeding. *These* people have older children and are moving into a new phase of parenting. *These* people may have protected rights and need certain considerations. Things have changed for *these* other people. It becomes intellectually and practically confusing for many people when boundaries start to become fuzzy. Dr Sally Dowling talks of liminality in the context of breastfeeding older children:

> Liminality comes from the Latin word 'limen' meaning a threshold. It describes when people are neither one thing or another. They are 'in between'. In our society, we understand when women are pregnant

> and when they are breastfeeding, but if they are continuing to breastfeed it becomes culturally confusing because they are not moving into the next stage.
>
> ~ (Dr Sally Dowling)

It may be that if you have read this far, it seems as though I am preaching to the choir. You may not feel you are someone who would ever say to a parent, 'Breastmilk is "just water" and has no benefit.' But I hope some of you are. We need the people who say 'There's no value now' and 'There's no need beyond six months' to care about their professional education in this area as they would in any other. And when a dentist said to Milda on hearing she was still breastfeeding her two-year-old, 'Does your GP know about this?', wouldn't it be awesome if the next line was 'I hope so, because they should know what a fantastic job you are doing!' They are likely to only get to that place with some additional education, beyond what was initially offered in their original degree and training, and a commitment to empathize with parents who may make decisions they don't entirely understand.

When it comes to supporting breastfeeding families with older nurslings, we ALL have to take a long, hard look at ourselves, otherwise known as professional self-reflection. The lactation consultant who breastfed until her child was three years old may not necessarily be better equipped to support the family of the five-year-old nursling than the professional who breastfed for three months or not at all. If you ask a group of passionate toddler-feeding parents when it starts to feel 'weird', they will often have their visceral limit as much as a group who stopped breastfeeding at four months. Whatever we don't have personal experience of can feel strange.

Daisy, breastfeeding Rex at three years and three months, breastfed his sister Gigi until she weaned during Daisy's pregnancy at 17 months:

> I remember a conversation I had with my husband once. We had been to a friend's son's one-year religious celebration and in the service he had toddled over to her and she had breastfed him. I was nine months pregnant with Gigi at the time. Anyway, roll on 15 months or so and I was feeding her and he said to me, 'How long are you going to feed her for?' I said I didn't know and asked him when he felt I should stop and he said, 'Well, as long as you aren't still feeding her when she is the same age as [our friend's] son.' I kindly pointed out that she was over that age already and he was so shocked. It's interesting how normalized breastfeeding had become to him that he hadn't recognized it in our daughter. Now with Rex, he doesn't even bother to ask.
>
> ~ *(Daisy)*

It can be all too easy to project our personal experiences onto the families we support. Intellectually, we know we are a wriggling mass of unconscious bias. It takes a vast amount of professional and personal skill to acknowledge those biases and work alongside them.

Many parents end their personal breastfeeding experience unhappily. In the UK, 80% say they did not breastfeed for as long as they wanted to. In the UK, nearly half of parents who initiate breastfeeding have stopped by six weeks and up to 90% report this wasn't their choice (Brown 2019, p.8). It appears that this is especially true of some groups of health professionals.

A 2013 study looked at the experience of 80 physician mothers (Sattari *et al.* 2013). Although the parental goal for duration of breastfeeding had been 12 months or more for 57%, only 34% of the children were actually still breastfeeding at 12 months. In 43% of cases, physician mothers stated that breastfeeding cessation was due to demands of work. Whether a physician parent continues breastfeeding directly impacts on their advocacy of breastfeeding in their working role.

> Mothers who did not continue breastfeeding after return to work were significantly less likely to report clinical (p=0.031) and workplace (p<0.001) breastfeeding advocacy... We did not find an association between physicians' clinical and workplace breastfeeding advocacy and maternal age, marital status, breastfeeding education (medical school or residency), partner work status, perceived level of support at work environment during pregnancy, length of maternity leave, duration of paid leave, maternity leave type, work schedule flexibility, infant feeding method at birth, maternal mental health postpartum, maternal energy level postpartum, maternal stress level postpartum, satisfaction with personal breastfeeding duration, availability of time or place at work for milk expression, and workplace support for breastfeeding efforts. (Sattari *et al.* 2013)

Research shows repeatedly that personal experience matters. In 1995, Freed *et al.* found that among a large national sample of physicians in training and practice, previous personal breastfeeding experience, or the experience of a spouse, was the greatest predictor of self-confidence in effective breastfeeding counselling (Freed *et al.* 1995).

On Facebook, there is the peer support group 'Breastfeeding for Doctors' specifically set up to acknowledge that doctors who breastfeed are in need of support, not least because if they do have a positive breastfeeding experience, the ripple effect on the parents they support throughout the rest of their career could be immense. If we take a moment to reflect on what it must feel like to be a health professional trying to support a breastfeeding situation when breastfeeding was virtually absent from your medical education, it is unfathomable. We have health professionals who are specialists in kidneys (nephrologists) and gums (periodontists). Where are the breast doctors? There are some cancer specialists who focus on breasts. There are some plastic surgeons who spend a large proportion of their career thinking about breasts. Where are the breast doctors who promote normal function of breasts, i.e. lactation? What about the doctors who understand hypoplasia (insufficient glandular tissue) or test prolactin levels as standard? The lactation specialists in our society are not medical by default but are often lactation consultants and breastfeeding counsellors coming from a lay background. IBCLCs (International Board-Certified Lactation Consultants) may sometimes be health professionals but there is no requirement for them to be one. Our medical school curriculums were shaped in decades past when breastfeeding rates were at their historical lowest, by people who didn't understand the science of breastfeeding nor its value to families. In a Norwegian study of GPs, only 26% could identify the differences between formula and human milk (Svendby *et al.* 2016).

> I'd say I totalled around one hour of breastfeeding education (through eight years' university education across two degrees, then a further five years' vocational training). The extent of the training was essentially 'breast is best' and I don't ever recall any mention of breastfeeding that wasn't in relation to a baby. I would say among GPs, the majority lack accurate knowledge about breastfeeding, especially beyond infancy. Non-evidence-based beliefs are very common, and often stem from their own negative breastfeeding experience. I'd go as far as to say that a large proportion of GPs believe that breastfeeding beyond infancy is weird and unnecessary. I'm thoroughly ashamed to say that those were my beliefs too, before I became a mum. I wasn't specifically taught this at university or during my vocational training, but I guess that this attitude arose out of ignorance and absorbing the culture I have grown up and live in.
>
> ~ *(A UK family doctor (GP))*

A UK study published in 2020 asked, 'Are the doctors of the future ready to support breastfeeding?' (Biggs *et al.* 2020). It collected data from 32 UK undergraduate medical schools and their students. The results showed that: 'A moderate ability to identify the benefits of breastfeeding was observed; however, self-rated confidence in practical skills was poor.' Only 3% of students felt that they had confidence in assisting with latching, which is the core skill of breastfeeding support at any stage. The research showed that 93% of students requested further breastfeeding education.

Imagine being a doctor, having received just a couple of hours in reference to lactation, and now in front of you is a family who feel breastfeeding is one of the most important elements in their lives. It is bound to be a challenge, and the vacuum left by insufficient medical education addressing lactation is understandably filled with personal experience and the experience of friends and family. The negative impact of this vacuum clearly affects the care families receive. Half of GPs and paediatricians in the UK advised families to introduce solids before the recommended six months in one study (Wallace and Kosmala-Anderson 2006). When families are inappropriately recommended to supplement with formula by paediatricians, it is more likely to lead to a complete end of breastfeeding (Taveras *et al.* 2004).

This is before we have even acknowledged the gaps in understanding breastfeeding that continues beyond six months and beyond 12 months. Quite simply, these families are often forgotten and professionals are often shocked when they meet a family breastfeeding an older child. When the Covid-19 vaccinations first started being offered in the UK, an early target population was professionals working on the front line of health care. Vaccine trials had not included breastfeeding parents, and in the absence of data, the vaccines were declared not appropriate for them. As is so often the case with breastfeeding and medication, absence of data was translated to mean 'unsafe'. The Infant Risk Center stated that:

> little or none of these vaccine components would ever reach the milk compartment, or even be transferred into human milk. Even if they were, they would simply be digested like any other protein by the infant. It is our opinion, that the present group of vaccines are probably going to be quite safe for breastfeeding mothers. The infant

may even gain a small amount of maternal IgG in the breastmilk, which may even be beneficial. (Hale and Krutsch 2021)

Problems started to arise when it became clear that working healthcare professionals were still breastfeeding, months or even years after a return to work. These professionals had previously been invisible to the regulators. It was only when a group of volunteers, including HIFN (Hospital Infant Feeding Network), GPIFN (GP Infant Feeding Network) and 'Breastfeeding for Doctors', gathered together and put pressure on them that guidance changed to allow parents to make their own decisions based on the lack of data. However, the damage was far-reaching, with many professionals ending breastfeeding prematurely or having to make a difficult decision about what to prioritize. Many involved in vaccinating did not receive the updated information and parents continued to be turned away well after the guidance was changed (*British Medical Journal* 2021 – see the second letter onwards). None of this would have happened in a society that valued breastfeeding, and valued breastfeeding older children sufficiently. For starters, breastfeeding mothers and parents would have been included in the initial trials.

With breastfeeding older children, the simple truth is we live in a world where breasts are seen as sexual. Some cultures do better than others at acknowledging their multi-purpose nature, but most of us grow up surrounded by the dominant message that breasts are private and something to do with sex. It's a challenge for the people doing the breastfeeding too. Throughout our lives, the mission has been to hide breasts away. We wear clothing that makes nipples invisible. We can buy small circular devices whose only purpose is to hide the shape of a nipple under clothing. We want bra straps to be secret. 'Sexy' people show their breasts in specific contexts, and other than that, the message is loud and clear that breasts are not part of discussion.

It's rare for breastfeeding and human lactation to be on the science curriculum at school. We potter along in ignorance for two or three decades and then suddenly when pregnancy happens, we're expected to do a 180-degree turn. Now, immediately, we're expected to understand that all that sexualization needs to be parked because breasts have a purpose. It's not hard to see why breastfeeding and breastfeeding in public isn't easy for everyone.

Breasts are often compartmentalized. The sexiness is supposedly switched off when maternity kicks in and it is assumed that sexiness may only resume once breastfeeding is controlled and ended. This is a challenge when we often live in societies where the nuclear family and the core couple is seen as central and a successful couple is a sexually active couple. Just as the breastfeeding parent struggles to reconcile being a parent alongside being a sexual partner, their spouse may too. It is not unusual to hear of parents 'wanting their body back' or partners 'missing' breasts. Those who continue breastfeeding for several years, perhaps even getting pregnant and having further children throughout breastfeeding, seem to have been able to break down the compartments and have breasts that can be both functional and sexual. A lactating breast is no barrier to a healthy sexual relationship and it may be that people's 'ickiness' at this concept is as much a barrier to accepting breastfeeding beyond the first few months as the visual of an older child at the breast.

If hearing about someone breastfeeding a five-year-old provokes a reaction in you, can you put your finger on why? That five-year-old grew older day by day. Parents don't often choose to breastfeed older children, they just choose not to stop. Ashley, feeding Bertie aged 24 months: 'It seemed a really alien idea just to stop when we had no reason to.'

We'll discuss later that there isn't evidence to suggest the milk loses immunological or scientific value. But even if it did, even if the purpose is for comfort, aiding sleep and relaxation, how does that make you feel? What about if the child had chronic eczema and asthma? Acceptable now? A serious cow milk protein allergy that triggers anaphylaxis? What about if the child had leukemia? What about if they were three and had a serious cow milk protein allergy or were two years old? What about if the milk was expressed with a breast pump and put in a cup? Where are your lines? We all have them and we all need to reflect on why we have them. Am I irritating you by asking these questions? You may feel you are entirely supportive of families and their feeding goals and have no lines, but I challenge you to acknowledge that you do and find out where they are.

Many of us who support families are also parents ourselves. Even if we are not, it's likely that we have parents who are close friends or family, and to state the obvious, we were all once parented ourselves. When we meet someone breastfeeding an older child, that may trigger something for us. It may go beyond the fact that this parent is breastfeeding when you perhaps did not, or for not as long. The fact they may appear to be centring their child implicitly feels like a judgement on those that don't. Their mothering or parenting is responsive and connected. They may appear to be making sacrifices that you either couldn't or didn't wish to or weren't able to. They might stay at home when you returned to work relatively quickly. It may not be the breastfeeding itself that feels uncomfortable but something deeper about their presentation of motherhood or parenting. It may be that individuals we are focused on supporting rub us up the wrong way and it's our job to try and consider why. They may remind us of someone else. If we don't understand the reasons why someone may continue to breastfeed on scientific grounds, we may add in some projection. It may appear self-indulgent. If you do not have experience of daily life feeding an older child, you may even perceive that feeding only continues because the parent is willing it.

It may be that you work in a setting where you associate longer-term breastfeeding with pathology. The children who seem to be hanging on to breastfeeding may have underlying health conditions and breastfeeding may then continue in response to pain and distress. It's an easy way to get nutrition into a child who lacks energy or who struggles to eat other food. When you meet a four-year-old who is breastfeeding, could it be that perhaps you are not hardwired to think of such children as normal and healthy because of previous professional experience in your medical field?

It may also be that we are put in a position of feeling more vulnerable because it is likely this client/patient is an expert in a way we are not. If we work in health, we want to make a positive impact and we've seen that it's unlikely your training will have thoroughly covered breastfeeding an older child. This parent may know a great deal more than you and it is a natural human reaction to fear ridicule or fear coming across as incompetent. Those who are devoted to this subject amass huge amounts of knowledge, and knowledgeable people can appear smug to those who feel threatened. When several of these elements come together, in our worse moments, we may even have an urge to 'take someone down a peg or two'. In our less worse moments, we may be conveying something in our micro-expressions and our tone of voice that we are not even aware of.

If you have an electronic device with internet access nearby, have a search for the *Time* magazine cover from May 2012. It has the text 'Are you mom enough?' and a mother is breastfeeding her older child who is standing on a chair to reach her breast. This cover was created to provoke reaction but it also provoked reaction in those who would consider themselves supportive of breastfeeding. How does it make YOU feel? She is beautiful by universal standards of beauty. She has her hand on her hip and is looking directly at the viewer. Her son is not wearing cute babyish clothes. He has camouflage trousers and a grown-up haircut. This is not a cuddly photo where he is tapping into his toddler instincts. This is a bloke who could step down from the chair and join in a game of football. She is absolutely unapologetic about the fact she is breastfeeding. Her priority is not your comfort levels. She has little time for your lack of training or lack of understanding. She will be unimpressed if you were to say anything negative about her breastfeeding experience. If she was to visit you about a medical issue unrelated to breastfeeding and her son was to latch on, how would you feel? What about if it was three years later and he was six years old? Would you flinch, even if just for a moment? Would you do more than that? Would you feel differently if she was less attractive, looked embarrassed, seemed disorganized, asked your permission?

Introduction

For some, the concept of feeding an older child provokes feelings of anger and even disgust. Dr Sally Dowling explains:

> When people don't understand that can move into frustration and almost anger. And there can also be disgust when we're talking about breast milk. There is a lot of anthropological thinking about how body fluids, particularly women's, are often seen as disgusting. An observation in a support group (published in a paper by Mahon-Daly and Andrews, quite some time ago now – 2002) (Mahon-Daly and Andrews 2002) noted that when formula milk was spilt it was cleaned up happily but when breast milk was spilt it was seen as disgusting in a completely different way. So some of the discomfort about breastfeeding older children could be coming from that place of disgust. Our bodily fluids, whether it's menstrual fluid or breast milk leaking, are often expected to be hidden and we struggle when they are 'out of place'. And perhaps breastfeeding an older child is breast milk 'out of place'.
>
> ~ *(Dr Sally Dowling)*

Breastmilk is often acceptable only in very restricted circumstances. It is permitted when a child is perceived as young enough and it is going directly into their mouth under a limited number of conditions. It quickly becomes disgusting for many when seen through leaked clothing, stored in a communal workplace fridge, posseted from a child's mouth or appearing during a sexual encounter. We need to reflect on where our own boundaries are and how they might differ from other people's and the families we care for.

Reflective practice is essential. It can't be a one-off, one activity on a training day, one piece of writing that confesses that, 'yes, breastfeeding a four-year-old does feel triggering for you because you unhappily gave up at 11 months', or it makes you feel as though your own parenting wasn't 'good enough'. It will be an ongoing process. You may look for supervisors or mentors who can help you think through your feelings and thoughts. Supervision may include increasing breastfeeding knowledge in some professional and voluntary settings but it should also be a place where your thinking is challenged. We want someone to ask the difficult questions. Have you ever not 'liked' a client? Ever felt your heart sink when they make contact? Why might they spark that reaction in you? How do you think they see you? Take five minutes to write about a consultation you had with a client who was breastfeeding an older child. You could use voice dictation on your phone or record yourself speaking. You might write by hand, not worrying about spelling and punctuation. Or write a list of adjectives or phrases. Read or listen to what you recorded. What strikes you?

How do you think a client would describe a session you just had? If someone you admire was watching a video recording of the session, what would they think? Would they feel anything was missing? We want those who are feeding older children to comfortably tell us they are. Do they return to you? Do they recommend you? Are they thankful for your support?

It's important to reiterate that personal breastfeeding experience is not a guarantee of easy acceptance of breastfeeding an older child, nor even the fact someone breastfed into toddlerhood. When you encounter a nursling who is four or five years old and your identity as a parent is strongly shaped by the fact you proudly breastfed until 18 months, you may have even more work to do. Breastfeeding support is often built on women supporting women but we live in a society where women are often pitted against one another and compared against one another. Your experiences may not always be positive. Judy Clinton (speaking about supporting women in general): 'I haven't had daughters or sisters, these women do still press the buttons of my school-day bullying by girls, which I'm aware makes me wary: I have to work harder to feel warm towards them' (Bolton with Delderfield 2018, p.38).

Often acceptance of breastfeeding older children simply comes from experience and exposure. Most of us live in a society where it isn't our normal. Every time we see an example of an older nursling, we change our hardwiring. In the context of her teaching around anti-racism, Nova Reid describes how it is possible to re-write our basic programming to undo prejudice (Reid 2020). It begins with acknowledgement that unconscious bias exists. It is not enough to claim allyship by claiming you are never overtly prejudiced in your actions and words. In the context of breastfeeding support, every time we see an older child breastfeeding or read an account of their experience, we can change our bias. It may mean looking for Instagram accounts or searching the hashtags #extendedbreastfeeding, #toddlernursing, #naturaltermbreastfeeding. You may even start a support group focused on those breastfeeding beyond 12 months, perhaps with a colleague who has more experience. Find ways to undo your unconscious bias.

We do have an immense responsibility. This is a population of parents who often feel very socially isolated. They may not know anyone who breastfeeds in real life. A few moments from a health professional may create memories that years later are told to someone like me:

> I had positive experiences when talking to healthcare professionals about still feeding him. He has eczema and an allergy to Brazil nuts. When I say he's breastfed, I normally get 'well dones' and encouragements.
>
> ~ (Sandra)
>
> At the ten-month developmental review, despite telling the health visitor that sleep was not an issue (I chose to be discreet about our actual sleeping arrangements which I now think was cowardly of me), she proceeded to plug some kind of gradual retreat sleep programme... I fully expected her not to understand or empathize with me as a breastfeeding mother who bedshares. Worse than that, I thought I might be reprimanded by her despite being happy and

comfortable with our arrangements. I came away feeling that I would not approach health visitors again for help or advice.

~ *(Hazel)*

During my second pregnancy, I told lots of midwives I saw that I was still feeding my 22-month-old, and without fail everyone was very positive and supportive about it. One midwife said she had tandem fed and her toddler had got a bit chubby!

~ *(Jo)*

I had previously had a very negative experience of speaking to health professionals when it came to problems with breastfeeding so I was extremely cautious of asking for help this time.

~ *(Sharon)*

At seven months, when Munch was diagnosed with food allergies, I was told it was my milk (that they had been drinking for the last seven months). Luckily, I knew differently as we have allergies in the family, but this misinformation has continued with the exception of our GP. When my child was two, I was told 'breastmilk is just water and has no benefit'.

~ *(Vanisha)*

My health visitor is a great supporter of extended breastfeeding so has always fully supported me. I'm currently 35 weeks pregnant so back seeing my midwife again and she has been great and supportive about tandem feeding if we are lucky enough to get that far.

~ *(Lucy)*

My GP was a little dismissive of my breastfeeding journey. When Arthur was sick at about ten months, they commented that I 'didn't need to still be doing that' or words to that effect. I found this to be

> disrespectful of my choices, and also inappropriate given I was there to discuss a chest infection.
>
> ~ (Lucy)

Families need support from professionals who understand why breastfeeding matters to them and why it is important to be able to continue if you want to. Breastfeeding an older child is far more than a milk delivery system. It is often a key parenting tool. It can't be switched off like a tap to take a certain medication or to have an operation, and if that is carefully researched and felt to be essential, the loss of breastfeeding may be felt profoundly.

You may have noticed that this topic is discussed as simply 'breastfeeding older babies and older children' so far. Terms like 'extended breastfeeding', 'natural-term breastfeeding' or 'long-term breastfeeding' have limited value. 'Extended' obviously implies 'beyond the normal', which is unlikely to make anyone feel good and also reinforces misconceptions that continuing to breastfeed is insignificant and not supported by evidence. Using the word 'natural' is rarely useful when discussing parenting and it is perhaps just as natural to wish to wean at 14 months and encourage your child to do so, as it is to breastfeed for several more years. Even long-term breastfeeding may not be helpful when someone's long-term is two years and another's is seven years.

When a term is absolutely needed to make a distinction, parents do seem to have a more positive association with 'natural-term breastfeeding' (Thompson, Topping and Jones 2020).

In one UK-based qualitative study looking at parents breastfeeding beyond 12 months:

> Women identified best with the term 'natural-term breastfeeding', explaining that breastfeeding beyond infancy is an aspect of biological heritage. All participants expressed dislike of the term 'extended breastfeeding' because 'it makes it sound not-normal', and

believed that the practice was perceived as 'extended' due to culturally imposed expectations: I believe in natural-term breastfeeding. (Thompson *et al.* 2020)

We will start with some assumptions. That we all understand that the current evidence-based recommendation is to breastfeed for around six months if you can, then introduce solid food alongside breastfeeding and to continue breastfeeding for two years and beyond. This is the recommendation of organizations as numerous as the World Health Organization, UNICEF, the American Academy of Pediatrics, the American Academy of Family Physicians, Health Canada, and the government health organizations of Australia, New Zealand and the UK.

It is not a recommendation just for people who live in countries with dirty water. As the *Lancet* series, examining breastfeeding in detail, pointed out in 2016, 'We estimate that an additional 22,216 lives per year would be saved by increasing breastfeeding duration from present levels to 12 months per child in high income countries' (Rollins *et al.* 2016).

Although the universal recommendations are well established, there is still confusion. The government of Northern Ireland has the phrase 'Breastfeed only for around six months, if possible' on its website in 2021 (www.nidirect.gov.uk/conditions/mastitis). A slightly unfortunate use of the word 'only'. It's interesting how the recommendation to exclusively breastfeed for six months is often half-remembered as 'breastfeed for six months'. Even those who have heard of the WHO-recommended 'two years and beyond' hear it as 'breastfeed for two years'.

What does 'and beyond' really mean? When is the stopping point?

Before we discuss breastfeeding beyond six months, let's celebrate getting to that point.

Chapter 2

Let's Celebrate Getting to Six Months and the Value in Continuing

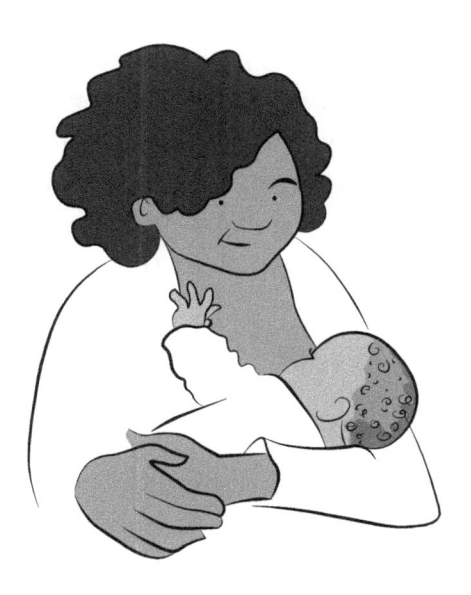

When we live in a society where only around 33% of babies are receiving any breastmilk at six months (UNICEF UK Baby Friendly Initiative 2021a), it can be difficult to celebrate breastfeeding achievements. When parents of eight- to ten-month-old babies were surveyed, 63% said they wished they had breastfed for longer (Renfrew *et al.* 2011).

There are a lot of disappointed families. The only space where parents may be able to talk about one of the most important achievements of their life is in a section of their social media life where they are surrounded by like-minded parents. They may not be able to voice their pride to close friends or family members as there is an agenda that the primary focus must be on not making others feel 'guilty'. We live in a world where marathon runners shout loudly, display medals and share their timings. I have yet to meet a marathon runner who keeps quiet on social media because there are some people who are physically unable to run a marathon and some people who once tried, but didn't succeed. How often do we hear from parents just how much feeding their child has meant to them?

> I am just incredibly grateful I am still breastfeeding my son. I have achieved degrees, led departments and lived on my own. But my largest achievement to date is breastfeeding. It has taken a lot of time, and literally blood, sweat and tears at some points, to get where we are. I am so grateful for being able to have access to breastfeeding support peers and groups such as Leicester Mammas who is still my vital form of support today.
>
> ~ (Meera)

Before we move on to discuss breastfeeding beyond six months, there must be space to acknowledge the achievement of reaching six months. In a flurry of busy days, this can too easily be forgotten. Health professionals who support families are uniquely placed. They are often in one-to-one consultations where the subject of breastfeeding is being raised. We often hear of stories of a mumbled 'Well done for getting to six months!' It can feel unnatural to offer praise to clients and patients. It may feel particularly odd if you believe breastfeeding is our default position as a species and you would no more praise someone for hugging their child. However, you may be the only person who acknowledges this milestone, and the strength and pride you can acknowledge in that parent not only validates what is often a tough six months but also will colour your future relationship with them and their ability to continue to share their journey with you.

Why was it worth it up until now? We can talk about nutritional and immunological benefits, the benefits to physical development and reaching IQ potential, impact on parental mental and physical health, relationship building, the impact on the environment and wider society. Of course, many would argue this is reversing the correct use of language. Instead we should be talking about the risk to babies who are *not* breastfed but that is not always appropriate when the choice to breastfeed is removed from parents by the lack of professional support and community support.

If we lived in a world where everyone chose to breastfeed freely, then discussing risk openly could be more comfortable. In reality, that would often mean talking about the risk of using formula with parents who had the choice removed from them. Antenatally, discussions of risk can be had more comfortably, but even then it is not always easy. We can start by looking at the impact on the baby who has been breastfed.

A baby is less likely to be hospitalized for vomiting and diarrhoea-related infections. There is often an assumption this is due to reduced exposure to pathogens. There is an assumption that the issue is drinking water which is sub-optimal or formula being made up incorrectly. Evidence is clear that breastfeeding has an impact in all nations, at all income levels regardless of the quality of your tap water and your ability to heat it up. The World Health Organization reminds us: 'Breastmilk contains several antimicrobial and anti-inflammatory factors, hormones, digestive enzymes and growth modulators that protect against infections' (Horta, Victora and World Health Organization 2013). Oligosaccharides are the third largest solid component of human milk and appear to change the way disease-causing pathogens behave in the infant gut, making it more difficult for them to adhere to mucosa. Human milk contains antibodies produced by parents once they have been exposed to pathogens. It contains factors that disrupt pathogens such as lactoferrin and lysozyme, breaking down cell walls, reducing inflammatory responses and preventing bacteria growth. This goes far beyond whether or not you are able to make up formula with clean water.

A 2010 study of 18,819 infants found that exclusive breastfeeding protects against hospitalization for diarrhoea. The researchers found that an estimated 53% of diarrhoea hospitalizations could have been prevented each month by exclusive breastfeeding and 31% by partial breastfeeding (Duijts *et al.* 2010).

There is reduced risk of a baby being hospitalized for a respiratory infection. Breastfeeding reduced the risk of hospitalization for respiratory infection by 57% (Horta *et al.* 2013).

It reduces risk of obesity. One study of 16 European countries suggests breastfeeding can reduce the risk of obesity by up to 25% (Rito *et al.* 2019).

The risk of SIDS (Sudden Infant Death Syndrome) is reduced. The Lullaby Trust in the UK states that: 'Breastfeeding for at least two months halves the risk of SIDS but the longer you can continue the more protection it will give your baby' (The Lullaby Trust 2021).

It reduces risk of some childhood cancers. A 2015 systematic review concluded, '14% to 20% of all childhood leukemia cases may be prevented by breastfeeding for 6 months or more' (Amitay and Keinan-Boker 2015).

It is associated with higher IQ scores and better educational attainment (leading to increased income). This has been found in studies which look at families from all social classes (UNICEF UK Baby Friendly Initiative 2021b). Professor Nigel Rollins in the *Lancet* breastfeeding series in 2016 described how 'Not breastfeeding is associated with lower intelligence and economic losses of about $302 billion annually or 0.49% of world gross national income' (Rollins *et al.* 2016).

It reduces the risk of ear infections. Using 2012 figures, £1.2 million per year would be saved in treating just ear infections if exclusive breastfeeding rates in the UK increased to 65% (Renfrew *et al.* 2012).

It reduces the risk of cardio-vascular disease (Owen *et al.* 2002).

A baby may have some protection against wheezing and asthma particularly when a parent has asthma. The evidence around asthma risk is less convincing than the evidence looking at other health conditions, but several studies show a protective effect. A 2011 New Zealand study showed: 'Breastfeeding, particularly exclusive breastfeeding, protects against current asthma up to six years. Although exclusive breastfeeding reduced risk of current asthma in all children to age six, the degree of protection beyond three years was more pronounced in atopic children' (Silvers *et al.* 2012).

A baby may have greater protection against developing type 1 diabetes (Patelarou *et al.* 2012).

Breastfeeding up to six months reduces the risk of dental malocclusion. A 2015 study found that: 'Those who were exclusively breastfed from 3 to 5.9 months and up to 6 months of age exhibited 41% and 72% lower prevalence of MSM (moderate/severe malocclusion), respectively, than those who were never breastfed' (Peres *et al.* 2015). Breastfeeding up to 12 months of age is associated with a decreased risk of tooth decay (Public Health England 2019). There is more on dental health in Chapter 3.

There are also numerous impacts that go beyond the immediate health of the child, parental health for one.

A 2017 study of 300,000 Chinese women found that 'a history of breastfeeding was associated with an ≈10% lower risk of [cardiovascular disease] in later life and the magnitude of the inverse association was stronger among those with a longer duration of breastfeeding' (Peters *et al.* 2017).

Breast cancer risk is reduced with a 4.3% reduction in invasive breast cancer risk with every 12 months of breastfeeding over a lifetime (Parkin 2011).

There is a reduced risk of developing type 2 diabetes. A 2018 study found:

Among young white and black women in this observational 30-year study, increasing lactation duration was associated with a strong, graded 25% to 47% relative reduction in the incidence of diabetes even after accounting for pre-pregnancy biochemical measures, clinical and demographic risk factors, gestational diabetes, lifestyle behaviors, and weight gain that prior studies did not address. (Gunderson *et al.* 2018)

Continued breastfeeding offers continued protection. A 2021 meta-analysis found: 'Each additional month of lactation was associated with a 1% lower risk of type 2 diabetes (RR 0.99, 95% CI (0.98, 0.99))', although researchers felt more studies were needed (Pinho-Gomes *et al.* 2021).

It has benefits for parental mental health. In a large UK-based study, the lowest risk for post-partum depression was among those who planned to breastfeed and were able to reach their feeding goals (Borra, Iacovou and Sevilla 2015).

It also benefits the environment. It is estimated that it takes around 4000 litres of water to produce 1kg of formula milk powder. In the USA, 550 million cans, 86,000 tons of metal and 364,000 tons of paper end up in landfill each year from formula packaging (Rollins *et al.* 2016).

There are also wider economic impacts for all members of society when breastfeeding rates increase. It means less investment needed in health care, greater productivity and a more efficient use of resources. Keith Hansen, from the World Bank Group, wrote in 2016:

> If breastfeeding did not already exist, someone who invented it today would deserve a dual Nobel Prize in medicine and economics. For while 'breast is best' for lifelong health, it is also excellent economics. Breastfeeding is a child's first inoculation against death, disease, and poverty, but also their most enduring investment in physical, cognitive, and social capacity. (Hansen 2016)

Those of us involved in breastfeeding support rarely use the phrase 'breast is best'. In her article 'Watch your language!', Diane Wiessinger reminded us that when breastfeeding or human milk is seen as superior and 'the best', the alternative is normal and adequate. In fact it is breastfeeding that is the norm and anything else misses out. I expect she would not be thrilled with the list above that describes the 'benefits of breastfeeding' or that breastfeeding 'reduces risk' (Wiessinger 1996). She reminds us that, 'When we talk about the advantages of breastfeeding – the "lower rates" of cancer, the "reduced risk" of allergies, the "enhanced" bonding, the "stronger" immune system – we reinforce bottlefeeding yet again as the accepted, acceptable norm.' As I mentioned, I followed the convention often employed in societies where breastfeeding rates are low and goals often not reached.

What is the evidence around the value of continuing to breastfeed beyond six months? Here is a time to put our foot down and say that for parents who wish to continue breastfeeding their child, the value is *that they wish to continue breastfeeding their child*. For every parent who is combing through the internet searching for evidence to justify their decision, there is someone challenging them who lacks an urge to research anything.

Like most professionals who support parents feeding older children, I am regularly contacted by families who are looking for ammunition in a battle to support their decision to continue. They embark on a journey already feeling on the wrong side of the power balance. It feels as though the people challenging them have science on their side and they must go down a rabbit hole of internet searches and trawling through scant research studies to justify something at the heart of their parenting. When someone says 'What are the benefits to continuing to breastfeed?' or another phrase that essentially means 'Prove it!', they are expecting parents to do the labour. The answers are too often dismissed if the resources are provided by lactation consultants or breastfeeding support organizations. I have often heard a version of 'They won't listen to someone like La Leche League. It has to be a reputable source.' Organizations that have been specializing in breastfeeding support for more than half a century can be dismissed in a single email, even if the resources they are citing contain peer-reviewed research from scientists at the top of their field. IBCLCs who provide a lengthy list of sources are 'not good enough'. The lines of judgement seem to shift mysteriously.

'Sealioning' is a useful 21st-century term here. On social media it refers to a harassment technique. The harasser politely asks for further evidence to support a view they are questioning. A provision of evidence is often followed up by another apparently civil request or a questioning of resources. The 'victim' is required to do the labour and the harasser is the one who has the power to assess sources and probe further. Further evidence is requested, and when the victim finally acquiesces and runs out of steam, the assumption is that they have failed to make their case. Sometimes these conversations are happening with family members. Family members who are living alongside a happily breastfeeding dyad can apparently have more faith in internet strangers than those they love with their lived experience. Sometimes these conversations are happening with professionals who are advocating for an end to breastfeeding.

We need to support parents to feel empowered to say, 'I feel the burden of responsibility is on YOU to look for evidence that breastfeeding should not continue.' The World Health Organization states clearly:

> Infants should be exclusively breastfed for the first six months of life to achieve optimal growth, development and health. Thereafter, to meet their evolving nutritional requirements, infants should receive nutritionally adequate and safe complementary foods, while continuing to breastfeed for up to two years or beyond. (World Health Organization, UNICEF 2003)

And no, Mr Sealion, nowhere does it say that this applies only to young children living in developing countries/lower income countries and not developed countries/higher income countries. It is also a common tactic to imply that extended breastfeeding is surely only relevant in settings where young children may struggle to get access to clean water and fuel to heat that water (to make up bottles of artificial milk) or a healthy varied diet. There is something ominous about the suggestion that children and families in other countries are 'different' by default, not least because it is dismissive of the poverty and hardship that exists in our own countries, even if these arguments were valid. Sadly, I do suspect that there may be discriminatory undertones in some assumptions around how families in other countries parent, as if it is baser to continue to breastfeed. Is a child who is attached to their parent throughout toddlerhood and into pre-school age somehow less sophisticated/advanced/cosmopolitan? Is it more 'scientific' or 'educated' to move away from breastfeeding at a younger age? Are assumptions being made about what parents who contribute to society should be spending their time doing? Is a parent who chooses to delay their return to the workplace to facilitate continued breastfeeding contributing less? A parent who chooses to breastfeed may sometimes be described as a hippy. What is the use of that word revealing? It suggests someone who is not part of the mainstream, who may make less economic contribution, or who is naive or unrealistic. What is the real meaning behind some of these assumptions aimed at parents who breastfeed older children? I suspect when we unpeel some of the layers, we may be shocked at what prejudices we are revealing. In reality, of course, it is continuing to breastfeed that makes a significant contribution to society and to the economics of our society. This is the decision that is scientific and advanced. There are countless organizations at the other end of the spectrum from 'hippy' that affirm its importance.

The American Academy of Pediatrics 'reaffirms its recommendation of exclusive breastfeeding for about six months, followed by continued breastfeeding as complementary foods are introduced, with continuation of breastfeeding for one year or longer as mutually desired by mother and infant' (American Academy of Pediatrics 2012).

The American Academy of Family Physicians: 'Health outcomes for mothers and babies are best when breastfeeding continues for at least two years. Breastfeeding should continue as long as mutually desired by mother and child' (American Academy of Family Physicians 2014).

The Academy of Breastfeeding Medicine ('a worldwide organization of medical doctors') (their website is www.bfmed.org): 'The average age at weaning ranges anywhere from six months to five years,' says Arthur Eidelman, MD, president of the Academy of Breastfeeding Medicine. 'Claims that breastfeeding beyond infancy is harmful to mother or infant have absolutely no medical or scientific basis... Indeed, the more salient issue is the damage caused by modern practices of premature weaning' (Breastfeeding Medicine 2012).

Two years and beyond is also supported by the health authorities in Canada (Public Health Agency of Canada 2020), Australia (Australian Government 2019), New Zealand (New Zealand Ministry of Health 2020) and the UK (NHS 2020).

It is sometimes hypothesized that the continuation of breastfeeding could have a negative impact on social development (sometimes replaced with the term 'independence') but this is not supported by the evidence. A study of children continuing to breastfeed in the Philippines looked at families with low incomes:

> The psychosocial scale used in our study is a predictor of abilities related to language acquisition, cognition, and psychosocial maturity deemed essential for primary school entrance and is also correlated with school readiness itself. Thus, our findings extend prior work to suggest that there may be benefits of breastfeeding to the domains of cognitive and psychosocial maturity that allow successful adjustment to school life in the primary grade levels. (Duazo, Avila and Kuzawa 2010)

An Australian study found a longer duration of breastfeeding was associated with positive mental health outcomes into adolescence:

> Breastfeeding for a longer duration appears to have significant

benefits for the onward mental health of the child into adolescence. Following adjustment of the associated socioeconomic, psychological and birth exposures in early life, breastfeeding for six months or longer was positively associated with the mental health and well-being of children and adolescents. (Oddy *et al.* 2010)

There is no evidence that a longer duration of breastfeeding is associated with separation anxiety or general anxiety. There is no evidence it is associated with ADHD or autistic traits.

In fact, research suggests the opposite and continued breastfeeding is associated with reduced incidence: 'After adjustment for several confounders, longer duration of breastfeeding was independently associated with better cognitive development and with fewer autistic traits' (Boucher *et al.* 2017). It should be noted that is not the same thing as saying 'breastfeeding reduces the chance' of some of these behaviours. The researchers from this 2017 study noted: 'we cannot rule out the possibility that infants who develop more autistic traits or ADHD symptoms during early childhood behaved in a way that incited their mothers to stop or reduce breastfeeding' (Boucher *et al.* 2017).

Breastfeeding longer is associated with positive speech outcomes such as earlier polysyllabic babbling. This is perhaps not surprising when we consider the motor skills that breastfeeding requires from tongue, jaw and surrounding muscles. Studies suggest that the neurological impact of breastfeeding also has a part to play (Vestergaard *et al.* 1999). One large US study of more than 22,000 children found that parents' concerns about their child's language and motor development 'generally decreased as breastfeeding continued >or=9 months', that is, those who retrospectively reported longer breastfeeding duration were less likely to report concerns later in their child's life (Dee *et al.* 2007).

We sometimes hear that nutritional benefits are 'lost' and this devalues breastfeeding. Again, this is not supported by the evidence. A 2020 study led by Dr Natalie Shenker from the Human Milk Foundation (and supported by the Parenting Science Gang community) studied breastmilk samples from a range of families breastfeeding babies and beyond. 'Our findings suggest remarkable consistency in human milk composition over natural-term lactation' (Shenker *et al.* 2020). This study concluded that donor milk banking can accept samples up to 24 months post-partum as 'we show that the macro-level metabolic and microbial composition of human milk is maintained between three and 24 months of nursling age, with variations in small numbers of metabolite features observed as the nursling age increases beyond 24 months'. There may even be 'a possible increase in overall fat content'. Further research is needed to look at longer-term breastfeeding.

There are significant nutritional benefits that continue past babyhood: 'Breast milk continues to provide substantial amounts of key nutrients well beyond the first year of life, especially protein, fat, and most vitamins' (Dewey 2001). Dewey calculates that a nursling who is aged 12–23 months and is consuming 448 ml of milk daily will receive 29% of their energy requirements, 43% of their protein requirements, 36% of their calcium, 75% of their vitamin A, 76% of their folate, 94% of their vitamin B12 and 60% of their vitamin C.

Of course, why would we expect any different? What makes logical sense in terms of evolution and human history?

Katherine Dettwyler has done some useful work comparing humans with their fellow primates. She reminds us that talk of a worldwide average age of weaning is not useful:

> One often hears that the worldwide average age of weaning is 4.2 years, but this figure is neither accurate nor meaningful. A survey of 64 'traditional' studies done prior to the 1940s showed a median duration of breastfeeding of about 2.8 years, but with some societies breastfeeding for much shorter, and some for much longer. It is meaningless, statistically, to speak of an average age of weaning worldwide, as so many children never nurse at all, or their mothers give up in the first few days, or at six weeks when they go back to work. (Dettwyler 1995)

What is useful is to look at the biology of humans and perhaps discover where natural weaning would lie in a culturally neutral environment.

Dettwyler looked at six comparisons:

1) The emergence of first permanent molars is often a time for weaning in primates. In humans, that's around six years old.

2) Chimpanzees and gorillas nurse for around six times the length of their baby's gestation. This puts us at around four and a half years.

3) Larger mammals nurse until their infant has quadrupled their birth-weight in many cases. This puts us at around two and a half to three and a half years.

4) Other primates nurse until their infant is a third of their adult weight. For humans, this is around five to seven years and boys would breast-feed for longer than girls.

5) Other non-human primates appear to wean at about halfway to sexual maturity (which may put us at around seven years).

6) The continuation of nursing until the full development of the immune system. This puts us at around six years. 'The fact that children's immune systems do not become mature until six years of age is understandable if we assume that the active immunities provided by breastmilk were normally available to the child until about this age.'

Dettwyler points out that this list could have gone 'on and on'. All this would put our natural weaning age between two and a half years and seven years.

Several of the immunological properties in breastmilk increase in concentration in the second year. This makes sense when you consider that this is when a nursling is going to become more mobile and is likely to come into contact with more pathogens. 'Human milk in the second year postpartum contained significantly higher concentrations of total protein, lactoferrin, lysozyme and Immunoglobulin A' (Perrin et al. 2017). Lysozyme breaks down the cell wall of bacteria protecting against infections like salmonella and E. Coli. Lactoferrin binds with iron which makes iron more easily metabolized and also prevents its use by pathogens, preventing infection. One 2019 study looked at lactoferrin into the 48th month and suggested: 'Evidence of stable or rising immunoprotein levels during prolonged lactation provides an argument for foregoing weaning' (Czosnykowska-Łukacka et al. 2019).

Increasingly, responsive parenting is being advocated as the norm. UNICEF Baby Friendly in the UK has embraced responsive parenting as the core of early parenting and we need to take these messages to their logical conclusion. As the conversation focuses more on close and loving relationships, the first 1000 days and infant and parental mental health, the idea that breastfeeding is limited to only the first few months appears increasingly incongruous. As Katherine Dettwyler says: 'an understanding of our primate heritage should help protect women from misguided charges that they are "infantilizing" their children and preventing their normal development into independent children by prolonging breastfeeding' (Dettwyler 1995). Studies of communities that may be described as traditional societies also point to a weaning age of between two and five years, with some examples exceeding six years (Dettwyler 1995).

The cultural noise that seeks to bury the message that longer-term breastfeeding is normal can be overwhelming. Breasts are commodities that are used as tools in advertising scores of products, and when breasts are for lactation, those messages are more likely to struggle.

It is also the case that the follow-on formula industry is gaining in its influence and this may mean the message that longer-term breastfeeding is normal will be hidden further. Experts predict that 'the follow on milk segment is predicted to witness the highest compound annual growth rate in the global market…during the forecast period (2020–27)' (Fortune Business Insights 2020). In the UK, the advertising of first formula for babies under six months is against the law, as the UK adopted themes from the WHO international code on the marketing of breastmilk substitutes (World Health Organization 1981) into legislation. This has rallied the industry to promote follow-on formula for use from six months in print, television and on social media. Everywhere is the message that parents will be 'moving on' from breastfeeding. The top-selling baby-milk manufacturer in the UK, which spends heavily on television advertising, had a market value in 2020 of £163.6 million. The second best-selling brand (owned by the same parent company) had a share of £102.2 million (Statista 2021).

The Scottish infant feeding survey indicates that use of follow-on formula after six months is widespread even though the position of the NHS is that first formula is suitable for the first 12 months. Nearly a quarter of those who introduced follow-on/second formula did so on the advice of a health professional (Scottish Government 2018). The most popular brand of formula in the UK works hard to reach out to health professionals. In 2021, the UK Baby Feeding Law Group published a document aimed at health professionals: 'Danone Nutricia: Why do they want to be your partner?' (Baby Feeding Law Group 2021). Studies have shown that health professionals are confused by the cross-promotion of formula products and parents are too. In one Italian study, only 43% of parents were able to assign a type of formula to the correct age bracket (Cattaneo et al. 2015).

Social media has connected parents who choose to feed their babies in the longer term but it has also provided opportunities for formula milk companies, and advertising regulations are struggling to keep up. In their 2018 analysis of the practices of formula companies, Save the Children commented that 'Twitter, Facebook, Instagram and other similar sites allow behavioural targeting of products in a way that was never possible in the first days of the Code' (Mason and Greer 2018). When a parent uses a UK government supported tool – the Start4Life breastfeeding friend on Facebook – it increases the targeted advertising they receive for non-breastfeeding-related products (as of March 2021; it is hoped this will change).

We may feel that Instagram has empowered parents to normalize breastfeeding beyond babyhood. Every day, searching with hashtags like #breastfeeding, #naturaltermbreastfeeding and #breastfeedingtoddler, you can find families sharing their lives. They look real and positive and many also look Instagram fabulous. However, companies with vast resources are not to be under-estimated and are primed to use the parent blogger and influencer to their advantage. The first generation of Instagram influencers, who rely on social media for their income and personal validation, are moving into parenthood. An Instagram pioneer with four million followers who originally gained her reputation by discussing cleaning became a mother and entered into a relationship with a bottle manufacturer, sharing discount codes and promoting products. In 2019, another UK-based influencer with 1.4 million followers used Instagram to promote a growing-up milk and posted herself bottle-feeding her 18-month-old on a sheepskin rug next to the fire with the formula container on the ground next to her. Formula companies are fully aware of the power of micro-influencers who are even more likely to operate under the radar when it comes to WHO code compliance. The 'breastfeeding beyond babyhood' industry has no comparative resource at their disposal. Social media is still struggling to understand how their restrictions around nudity sit alongside an acceptance of breastfeeding, and in 2021, breastfeeding-related posts are still being restricted and removed, often by algorithms and bots rather than real people.

Who might pay for any kind of campaign around longer-term breastfeeding? When most health services are under-resourced and focused on trying to improve breastfeeding initiation and supporting parents getting to six weeks, let alone six months, there isn't an obvious answer. The Canadian government put out a campaign in 2013. One image says 'Breastfeeding is not just for newborns' as a toddler latches on (Velez 2013). However, where most parents will encounter such an image is in an internet search trying to find evidence that there has ever been a public health campaign supporting breastfeeding older children.

There are families living in Western societies who are surrounded by a dominant culture that may not value continuing to breastfeed but have their own motivations for wishing to continue based on their family's cultural and religious background. There may be strong cultural support despite other barriers such as limited access to specialist care or a pressure to return to work quickly (Steinman *et al.* 2010).

Breastfeeding beyond babyhood has a special significance in Islam (Bayyenat *et al.* 2014). The Quran says (in translation) that 'the mothers shall give suck to their children for two whole years'. It is perceived as the right of the child to be able to breastfeed for these two years. Although it is also when the parents desire it and when it is possible, rather than something that should be a burden. The Federal National Council in the United Arab Emirates went as far as proposing a clause in a child rights law that breastfeeding should be mandatory for the first two years and this was passed into legislation in 2014 (Constantine 2014). There is a difference of opinion on what happens after two years, however. This is something that an individual will find their own answers to if religion is central to their life, rather than something a non-Muslim lactation consultant has a right to dictate the final word on. Some traditional narratives and interpretative scholars make it clear that up to 30 months is supported by scripture, or even to the end of the third year, but not beyond that. Some will suggest that an absence of specifics means a parent will decide for themselves.

The final word will rest with parents. If they feel it is right for them and their child to continue to breastfeed, it is the responsibility of professionals and wider society to support them. Science, history and economics are on their side. It's also important to note that for many families, continuing to feed an older child just happens. It may not be something that they set out to do. In fact, research suggests that few parents make the decision antenatally to feed beyond infancy but it develops as a natural progression. A qualitative study from 2020 reported:

> All of the women had planned to initiate breastfeeding, but had not intended to breastfeed beyond one year at the time of their first

pregnancy. Instead, participants readjusted their breastfeeding intentions as children grew. Many of the women reported that they had not been aware of the recommendations regarding breastfeeding duration antenatally, and had been unaware it was possible to continue to feed an older child. (Thompson *et al.* 2020)

Many parents themselves start out with the prejudices shared by wider society. They may even have been disgusted or horrified at the thought of breastfeeding an older child, but their personal experience and their desire to meet the needs of their child changed their views. Their exposure to the reality of an older child breastfeeding brought about a shift. Perhaps we will see a cultural shift in society the more the wider population are exposed to natural-term breastfeeding as normal.

> Positives are that I'm so proud I've been able to continue and bring quick comfort for my son beyond six months. He is such a settled soul and I like to think that's been helped by continuing to successfully breastfeed. Personally, as I have multiple sclerosis, I believe that the health benefits for the mum from breastfeeding has helped keep me well and relapses at bay. My only small regret is how he only seems to settle with me easily, but that regret is not significant enough to stop feeding at this stage.
>
> ~ *(Kim Frost)*
>
> There is no way Nina was ready to stop breastfeeding after six months. I truly believe it would have had a very negative impact on Nina if we took this away. The calming nature of feeding alone was needed let alone the countless health benefits. Both of us have researched the long-term impact of continuing feeding and we want this for our daughter. Maira and I both agreed early on that attachment is one of the most important aspects of early parenting, breastfeeding plays such an important role in this. It's still clear to see how calm and

> secure Nina feels when she is feeding. Nothing else has that effect on her. If she feels unwell or hurts herself it's still the best thing for her.
>
> ~ *(Toby Walsh, dad to Nina, 20 months)*

For parents

As you reach six months and go beyond it, it can be valuable to pause for a moment and find some space for reflection and recording. These few months have been a significant moment in your life and your child's life. You may want to look back on these reflections by yourself or share them with your nursling when your breastfeeding journey comes to an end. You may share them one day when your child is a parent themselves.

- What are your memories of your first breastfeed?
- What has been the hardest aspect of breastfeeding?
- What has been the most rewarding aspect?
- How do you feel about reaching six months?
- What helped you to reach six months?
- As you continue, who will be supporting you? Is there more information you need? What will be changing?
- How would you describe your breastfeeding goals?
- What would you like to say to your breasts, your body?

Chapter 3

Conversations with Others and the Role of the Partner

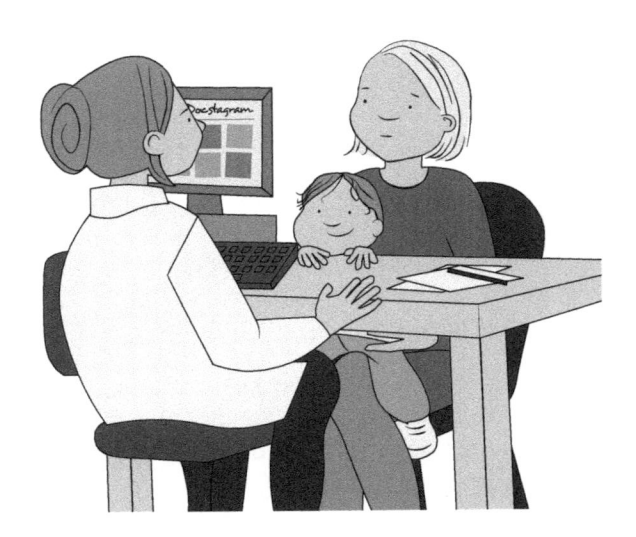

Although parents breastfeeding older children may feel like they are in their own little world, we are social animals and conversations with others in the community cannot be under-estimated in the way they affect us. They can boost us in the hardest moments and undermine our confidence in the worst way. There isn't a way to beat around the bush here. Parents who breastfeed beyond six months are repeatedly talking about negative experiences in their conversations with others. Some of us may be lucky enough to live in cultures and communities where breastfeeding older children is celebrated and recognized. Many of us are not. Many of us live in societies where the majority of people don't reach their breastfeeding goals. In the USA, the figure is around 60% (Odom *et al.* 2013). This can mean that parents who choose to continue to breastfeed are often tip-toeing around the trauma of others. There are few places where parents feel they can celebrate their breastfeeding achievements, or even talk about them openly. Some parents are literally fearful of talking about their continuation of breastfeeding. They may fear the involvement of social services or child services if they are discovered to still be breastfeeding, although social services should understand that continuing to breastfeed is not associated with abuse or neglect.

We live in a world where breastfeeding is often understood to be the ideal way to feed a baby, but that message isn't always backed up with practical support, nor practical support for the professionals who are supposed to be supporting you. Specialist lactation support may not be available in your area or it may come at a cost. Parents may be surrounded by family members who parented in a generation where breastfeeding was not the norm and normal infant and toddler behaviour was poorly understood. They may have access to health professionals with minimal or no training in breastfeeding support. As time goes by, and their breastfeeding continues, parents often see their new parent buddies drop away. We may hear them say things like 'There were two of us left from our original group, now it's just me. I'm the only one still breastfeeding.' Or 'I don't know anyone else in real life who is still breastfeeding.'

We must take great care that just because it may not be 'typical' to breastfeed an older child, that does not mean it equates with it not being 'normal'. 'Physicians should be able to provide parents with complete and accurate information about "normal" breastfeeding and weaning practices in humans' (Dettwyler 1995). In reality, a shorter duration of breastfeeding is not normal when compared to other primates of our size, nor normal when looked at with a cross-cultural perspective.

The person a breastfeeding parent is likely to speak to most about their feeding experience is their partner if they are in a relationship:

Fi has been essential and I couldn't have done it without her. She encouraged me when no one else did. She helped me feel that I could carry on, despite the challenges, and that I could do it. She made things easy for me by managing other tasks, such as cleaning or cooking, so I could focus on resting and breastfeeding. Fi made it clear that she was not jealous of my ability to feed our children and that she was proud of me for doing it; she came up with her own ways of bonding with the girls and never once suggested she should bottle-feed (she did give a bottle of expressed milk a couple of times and she enjoyed the experience, but she treated it as an exception and never said it should be the norm).

Partners are absolutely vital to breastfeeding; they can research, verbally cheer you on, take responsibility for the household and childcare, ensure you are well fed and as rested as possible, and just generally make it so that the breastfeeding parent can make feeding the priority. Fi did all that for me and it made me love her even more than I already did, which I hadn't realized was possible.

~ *(BJ Woodstein, speaking about her wife)*

My husband and I didn't ever particularly discuss breastfeeding beyond infancy. It was a situation that just naturally evolved and came to be. I would say he quietly supported me in a fairly minimalist fashion. He wasn't shouting from the rooftops about me breastfeeding, but if anyone questioned/challenged it then he would show his support then by explaining that it was working well, there were no good reasons to stop, etc. Both of our families thought we were odd. Particularly my in-laws, who didn't breastfeed their children at all. My mum breastfed my brother and me but stopped when we were both babies. I've talked extensively to her about her breastfeeding experiences, and whilst she was happy with what she achieved at the time, she now feels (with the knowledge that I've passed on to her) that she would have breastfed for longer had she known more at the time. Both of our families got used to me breastfeeding and it was a topic for discussion. I feel like I've achieved a lot of education for them and normalization of breastfeeding – which I'm really proud of. I'd say I felt quietly supported by my parents when I had taught them information about the benefits of breastfeeding beyond infancy.

~ *(Naomi Dow)*

My husband, although completely supportive of breastfeeding, wasn't able to offer actual guidance or support, as he was completely new to this as well. But whenever I talked about breastfeeding beyond the first few months, he was always fully open and committed to it. He really likes the motto 'my body, my baby, my choice'.

~ *(Millie)*

My husband was quite instrumental in my breastfeeding journey. His support was great. I remember a conversation around the time Nicola was about six months old. I was breastfeeding her and he said, 'Just look at her, that's all you!' And I looked, quite puzzled, at him. He said, 'It is all your feeding and your breastmilk that is solely responsible for her growing and look what a gorgeous baby she is.' I never thought about it that way. To me, breastfeeding was the most natural thing to do without any thinking or any reason behind it. I was so proud of us.

~ *(Miriam)*

If a family is still breastfeeding after the first few months, and into the second year, the chances are that the breastfeeding parent's partner has been a team player.

What does a supportive partner look like?

> Pretty simple really. Just be there. Be available to talk through things and listen to how Maira feels, not to offer advice. Mostly listen. I always try to encourage when Maira is struggling. Right from the start I realized that my job was to take care of Maira while she took care of our daughter. I felt like a bit of a spare part for much of the first year as all Nina wanted was her mum. Nina now adores me and thinks I'm awesome, which is great for my ego, but she still goes to Maira when she wants to feel secure.
>
> I am there to do the things that Maira can't because she has a toddler attached to her. Mostly [it] is fetching things out of reach and saying how awesome Maira is and telling her how proud I am of her to keep going through all the struggles. I think it's safe to assume that without a supportive partner many families would not be able to continue with breastfeeding. I can remember a number of occasions when people have said things to Maira about how much she breastfeeds Nina or that she doesn't put her down enough and that the baby needs to learn to be put down. I always told them to mind their own business and reassured Maira that we are doing the right thing. I am there for Maira when she needs me but always do my best to be there before she needs me too if that makes sense.
>
> ~ *(Toby, supporting his wife Maira who is breastfeeding at 20 months)*

There is a special quality in a non-breastfeeding parent who can step back for a moment to give space to the connection that develops between a nursing pair. It is insulting to claim that dads and partners 'get jealous' when they see a special relationship develop, but it is inevitable that at times they may feel less needed and will look for ways they can offer value in those moments. These are families who worked out early on that the idea the non-breastfeeding parent should give a bottle to 'bond' with their child is about as daft as it sounds. For a mainly breastfeeding child, a bottle is not an equivalent experience and not a substitute for skin-to-skin contact and cuddles. They can be milk delivery systems, but it is the cuddles afterwards or before that bring the magic. The nursing relationship is the first intimate relationship, and partners who facilitate that, to the benefit of both their child and co-parent, are helping to bring positive mental and physical health impacts to everyone concerned. There may also be less lofty reasons why partners encourage breastfeeding to continue on occasion.

> From 12 to 24 months they fed usually between one and three times a day. My partner actively encourages them to feed, so he can get precious extra minutes in bed in the mornings on weekends, and so we can have some quiet moments on the sofa in the afternoons. He plants the idea in their head so he can have a break!
>
> ~ *(Rhian, who is feeding her 26-month-old twins after exclusively breastfeeding them in infancy)*

It sounds as though he has earned that right, as Rhian explains his role in their early breastfeeding journey:

> He was absolutely crucial to the success of our breastfeeding journey... We fed to sleep until 18 months and my partner was there almost every night to move the babies off the feeding pillow and into their cots once they were asleep. He was a pro at moving babies without waking them!
>
> ~ *(Rhian)*

For many non-breastfeeding partners, there seems to be every reason to continue. In rare cases, it may be them who is encouraging nursing to continue when the breastfeeding parent may be less sure. As breastfeeding supporters, we are so used to encountering the opposite that this can be a surprise. The breastfeeding parent may be co-sleeping and feeding several times a night. The nursling is thriving but the parent is beginning to look forward to an end to breastfeeding. They may be working outside the home alongside breastfeeding, experiencing aversion or just feel ready to move on. When the nursling is so clearly benefiting, it can be difficult to admit that you want to stop. If you have spent so long defending continuing to breastfeed, it may be that your partner struggles to empathize when you do want to bring it to an end. Perhaps you have been promoting the World Health Organization message of 'two years and beyond' so effectively that when you have reached 21 months, and you want to stop, your partner may not be on board. As Toby explained earlier, this is about listening and supporting.

Of course, some breastfeeding parents are in unsupportive relationships. There may even be cases where continuing to breastfeed felt like a catalyst for the end of a relationship. Truthfully though, it was representative of wider issues: a partner struggling to empathize with another, lacking respect for their feelings and what matters to them, feeling resentful of other relationships that offer joy and love and comfort. A partner that does not support you to achieve something that feels like it is at the heart of who you are and how you parent is not acting in partnership. In Chapter 8, on problems and challenges, we will discuss further when separation occurs in a family continuing to breastfeed. Breastfeeding parents who are single, whether from earlier on or from when a nursling is older, can be bombarded by the message that a new family is only 'functional' if it consists of two adults. Of course, this is not the case. Many single parents who breastfeed are among the most empowered and thriving as they make decisions that suit them and their child.

What about wider family members?

> I was lucky to have a huge amount of support from one family member whose voice I could listen to and trust among the barrage of (what felt like quite hostile) family breastfeeding opinions. She had fed several children herself, and would send me up-to-date information to give me the confidence to continue. She also pinpointed me to several online breastfeeding blogs that I could follow for support and I would have conversations with her that increased my confidence and enabled me to keep going. We would talk about the proven benefits of long-term breastfeeding for mother and child, as well as the amazing ways continued breastfeeding can help in everyday situations (like soothing an older baby or child when hurt, or instantly calming a toddler meltdown). In fact I've often felt that if it wasn't for her, I would have caved to the pressure to stop feeding long ago.
>
> ~ (Millie)

It is stating the obvious but there is enormous variation in what support parents can expect from their elderly relatives. During the Covid-19 lockdowns in the UK, parents continuing to breastfeed described very different feelings about their lack of contact with wider family. For months at a time, families with young children were unable to meet up with grandparents. In some areas, there was an option for families to meet on Christmas Day (though not everywhere) and there was a spike in anxiety for some parents who realized they might have to reveal they were still breastfeeding to family members who they knew to be resistant and unsupportive. Lockdown meant that nursing dyads could continue as they wished. Parents were often working from home. Partners were around. There was very little social contact with non-family members and zero inside the home. If breastfeeding continued, few people would even know, let alone express an opinion. It also felt sensible to continue in a world where a virus was a threat and a parent was producing a tool known to fight viral threats. At the other end of the spectrum, some breastfeeding families were missing their mentors. They knew they could ordinarily rely on grandparents to offer support alongside continued breastfeeding, tandem feeding and trying to find time to work while also caring for a demanding breastfeeding toddler.

A 2016 systematic review looked at the impact of grandmothers on breastfeeding. They found in the studies they looked at that:

> the overall effect on breastfeeding was positive when the older female generations' attitudes towards, or experiences with, breastfeeding was favourable towards breastfeeding. A grandmother's positive breastfeeding opinion had the potential to influence a mother [to such an extent that she is] up to 12% more likely to initiate breastfeeding. Conversely a negative opinion has the capacity to decrease the likelihood of breastfeeding by up to 70%. (Negin *et al.* 2016)

The researchers point out that the logical conclusion of this is that antenatal education should include older family members but cross-generational health education is rare. They suggest, 'The lack of attention to mothers-in-law in global health fits in to a larger reality of the neglect of older adults by the global health community' (Negin *et al.* 2016).

If we are going to support breastfeeding, and breastfeeding older children, we need to take a moment to consider the grandparents: both the highs and the lows of contact with grandparents. In breastfeeding support, particularly if home visits are our norm, we meet a lot of grandparents. Like many, I meet the ones who make an excuse to get me into the kitchen and it turns out they're not a cup-of-tea pusher (as many are) but they desperately wanted a moment to talk about their own breastfeeding experience. It was decades ago – usually 30 years plus – but there's an emotional mother in front of me and she's not the one I was expecting to be trying to help. She might be worried about her daughter or grandchild but often she's reflecting on her own mothering experience and she wants to share. She might want to tell me that she didn't breastfeed at all and she needs me to know that. Sometimes she's filled with regret: 'I wish I knew someone like you when my babies were small' is a common phrase. Sometimes she's angry about the lack of support she received. I've even had anger about the lack of support she received from her OWN mother.

When we support a parent, we are shaping a future grandparent too. One day they might be cornering someone in a kitchen. What will they say? Will they be filled with sadness, angry that the local breastfeeding group got cut, angry about the lack of midwife visits? And we're making the great-grandparents too. The gaps in support now will be felt for generations. And when support is there for new parents, we are helping an infant who may not be born until the next century.

It takes a great maturity to own your own regret, appreciate what happened to you and how YOU were failed and move on to be the kind of grandparent needed for a new generation. It's an enormous ask. And how much easier it is when a parent was able to reach their own breastfeeding goals and breastfeeding is a fond memory, not a space for feeling awful.

The grannies I meet in kitchens sometimes thought all was well. They didn't realize they DID regret anything. Feeding their child was a very long time ago, and it's only when they are suddenly faced with seeing breastfeeding again that a surge of emotions has taken them by surprise. Sometimes we know that surge can lead grandparents in unhelpful directions. It's a natural instinct to want to protect yourself. It's natural to want validation that what you did was 'the right way'. How you chose to parent is at the heart of who you are as a person. And after a long time, you might have forgotten that perhaps you didn't always get to choose how you fed your baby. Was it their choice when their healthcare professional told them to only breastfeed every four hours, or not to breastfeed at night, or to keep their baby in the hospital nursery for hours at a time? They were sabotaged, but they may not have realized it at the time. They may not be conscious that trying to lead a new parent down the same path is another act of sabotage.

Now, different choices are being made. There's this thing called 'responsive feeding'. The cot is hardly used. No one seems to mind when baby feeds again after only an hour. The baby hardly gets put down. The baby is still breastfeeding as more months go by. That can all feel very alien. It can also feel like an implicit criticism of the first few weeks, months and years they spent parenting. It takes a special person to take a pause and acknowledge that some of your struggles might be because of your need to validate your own mothering or parenting choices. If they didn't breastfeed at all, they naturally want to believe that their children are healthy. Someone told them not to 'spoil' their baby and they believed them, and it feels uncomfortable to imagine they might have been misled.

When a grandchild continues to breastfeed as the months and even years go by, there may be some projection going on. A grandparent may worry that their child's relationship with their partner will be impacted or it is bad for parental health ('You are exhausting yourself'). They may be sensitive to the fact that they live in a society where feeding older children is not the norm and worry that their child will encounter prejudice. They may worry that their grandchild will encounter prejudice at nursery or when starting school.

Incidentally, it is a common theme among social media and real-life discussions that starting school while breastfeeding is going to be a problem. Some parents fear a group surrounding their child in the playground taunting them for a mention of breastfeeding and that life-long bullying might follow. In my 25 years of experience as a breastfeeding supporter, parent and primary school teacher, I have yet to encounter an example of a child having difficulty when starting school as a long-term breastfeeder. The only example closely related was when a child requested a breastfeed in the playground at the end of the day and the teacher felt uncomfortable and expressed concern. Nothing ever followed from that. Children are forgiving and accepting and often exceed the expectations of adults. Truthfully, it is not something nurslings tend to discuss. They may already have picked up on the fact that it isn't always a topic that is discussed everywhere with everyone or they would no more go around shouting about it than they would announce loudly that their parents read them bedtime stories.

Grandparents may start out as supporters of breastfeeding but struggle more as time goes by. Encouragement turns into pursed lips and eventually negative comments may begin. Hopefully, by this stage, the nursing parent is equipped to manage the situation rather than suffer in silence. It may come down to education. It may come down to an open request to support their parenting choices or, at the very least, no longer talk about their feelings around this subject. There should be a simple rule that is a version of the common expression: 'If you can't say something nice, don't say anything at all.' If breastfeeding an older child is beyond someone's understanding, sometimes it is best to just remain quiet on the subject. Parents need to feel empowered to continue, and released from the responsibility of convincing others. They have no duty to provide a general education to those around them. Some days they may feel up to the task, but it is also to be encouraged when they step away from conversations, for reasons of self-protection.

Does any grandparent want to end up being a grandparent who is best sometimes avoided? Does anyone want it to be a potential silver lining of a pandemic that their grandchild could continue breastfeeding away from them as long as they wanted to? The grandparents who are supportive are an untapped resource. We need them to speak at community centres, make Instagram and TikTok videos and find their peers in the community who need to further their understanding.

It may not be the parents who are the only ones having challenging conversations. We sometimes hear reports of the nurslings themselves being approached by extended family members. There may be whispered comments like 'You're a big boy now. Why are you still having milk?' Disapproval may be conveyed with body language and facial expressions. Whether this is something a parent discusses openly with the nursling is a very individual decision. For older children, we are touching on areas that are crucial to their understanding of their right to body autonomy and their wider human rights. We are also giving them their first experience of dealing with family conflict and understanding how it is possible to disagree with someone you love and stand up to someone who you perceive as having greater authority. We may want to model conversations with them, help them explore what they want to say and make it clear that they are not alone. We may not always be there to protect them from the comments of others, though we can try.

As we have discussed, few health professionals address breastfeeding beyond infancy in their training. Even some lactation consultants, especially if they come from a health professional background, may be lacking in experience, though lactation consultants are likely to quickly get up to speed as they spend time immersed in the breastfeeding community and updating their professional learning. Conversations with health professionals can be some of the most significant conversations that parents continuing to breastfeed beyond infancy experience. Sadly, there are often negative experiences when parents are already feeling isolated and vulnerable. It can feel like a surprise when you make the natural assumption that someone devoted to public health would be a warrior in their support of breastfeeding.

> When my daughter was eight months old or so I went to the weighing clinic to check Kit's weight and I also wanted to ask how I would know she was getting enough milk given that she was eating some solids too; that question wasn't actually answered, but instead I was questioned about whether she slept through the night, which of course she didn't, and told she should be, and I should feed her a heavy meal before bed so she slept. At the time I was gob-smacked that I'd been given advice about something that I didn't have a concern with. When I look back on it, it was terrible that the straight advice about an eight-month-old baby is that he/she should sleep through. Such old-fashioned advice that is not protective of breastfeeding at all.
>
> After this experience, I made a complaint about it because I felt that the health visitor, while she was trying to help, was out of line and was giving out old-fashioned information that was not in line with WHO, GP Infant Feeding Network, UNICEF, etc. After this, I pretty

much avoided speaking to health visitors. That said, if I had to speak to one for any reason I would always drop in that my daughter was breastfeeding. I wanted it to be a more mainstream thing to hear. Or maybe I wanted them to challenge me so I could inform them.

When Kit was almost two, I visited a GP about getting on birth-control tablets. I'd done some research and wanted the mini-pill. When there, I told the GP that I had researched and wanted the mini-pill as I'd heard the combined could affect milk production because of the oestrogen. She scowled at me, asked me why I was still feeding. I was stunned and dumbly replied 'because she asks for it', to which I was told there was no benefit after six months. I sort of regained my composure, told her, 'Anyway, I'm not here to discuss breastfeeding', and eventually got my prescription. I made a formal complaint about this GP, which is still pending at the moment with the PHSO (Parliamentary and Health Service Ombudsman, who deal with NHS-related complaints).

~ (Carly)

The World Breastfeeding Trends Initiative (WBTi) team in the UK audited health-professional training in 2016. The WBTi is a tool that enables countries to assess their progress in breastfeeding and target resources more effectively. In many countries, the process is led by a collaborative team of government and third sector organizations. About 100 countries have already taken part. The UK report in 2016 asked whether health professionals were trained in areas such as the process of milk production and removal, the management of common feeding problems, the benefits of optimal infant feeding and prescribing medications compatible with breastfeeding. They concluded:

Most pre-registration training for healthcare professionals who work with mothers, infants and young children (midwives, nurses, health visitors, paediatricians, GPs, obstetricians, dietitians, pharmacists, maternity support workers) has many gaps in relation to the WHO education checklist in high-level standards and curricula. Where there are many gaps, the breastfeeding knowledge included tends to be theoretical rather than the practical aspects of enabling mothers to initiate and continue breastfeeding. (World Breastfeeding Trends Initiative 2016)

Change does not always come quickly and is so often led by individual champions rather than organizational drive. They may have had to pay for their own training or request their own training in the face of resistance. They may constantly feel as though they are fighting a battle for breastfeeding to be recognized – let alone breastfeeding beyond six and 12 months. Some of those individual champions may well be reading this. You are seen, and on those difficult days, every family you support is grateful. History and science is on your side (which may not be much comfort when you are trying to explain to your boss for the third time why the IBCLC exam is worth you doing). This is a difficult line to walk. By discussing the challenges parents face are we 'health-professional bashing'? Perhaps sometimes, yes. That is not the same as criticizing individuals but criticizing the system that pushes a nurse out into a world where she is expected to support families to use a breast pump without having a basic knowledge of how a breast pump works.

> I remember once a nurse coming to me saying a breast pump wasn't working because she couldn't feel suction against the palm of her hand. This is something you would do to test suction for a device used orally but she didn't realize you wouldn't expect the skin on the palm of your hand to pull into the pump.
>
> ~ (A hospital paediatrician from the UK)

Just as we talk about grandparents needing to resist the urge to be self-protective and centre their own experiences, the same is true of professionals supporting families. If your instinct is to respond with 'There are bad apples but most doctors/midwives/nurses are great', you are being dismissive. Breastfeeding beyond infancy is simply not in the curriculum in the vast majority of cases and families suffer as a result. Professionals also suffer as they are left in vulnerable positions and lack the resources to offer effective care to their clients and patients.

Parents breastfeeding beyond six months do report that conversations with dentists can be among the most challenging conversations they have with health professionals. On a surface level, this is perhaps not surprising. This is a group of professionals who come across children suffering with severe dental problems and, at the same time, they may have little or no training in breastfeeding and lactation. Breastmilk enters the body through the mouth. It contains 'sugars'. You can see how links end up being made: '[Breastfeeding] was not even mentioned, not once. We were taught to advise parents to stop all milk at night after the first year to avoid bottle caries' (Richa Sharma, a general dental practitioner in the UK).

Speaking on behalf of the UK government, Public Health England published a statement, updated in 2019, stressing the importance of dentists supporting breastfeeding and providing evidence-based care. They state:

> Breastfeeding is the physiological norm against which other behaviours are compared; therefore, dental teams should promote breastfeeding and include in their advice the risks of not breastfeeding to general and oral health... Since 2001 the WHO has recommended that mothers worldwide exclusively breastfeed infants for the first six months to achieve optimal growth, development and health. Thereafter, they should be given nutritious complementary foods as breastfeeding continues up to the age of two years or beyond. These guidelines were reiterated in the WHO's Global Strategy (World Health Organization, UNICEF 2003) and endorsed by the

Scientific Advisory Committee on Nutrition (SACN). (Public Health England 2019)

The evidence that breastfeeding up to 12 months is protective of dental health is well established, or to re-word: that *not* breastfeeding increases risk of dental caries. Breastmilk, unlike formula, contains Lactobacilli, human casein and secretory IgA among other substances, which inhibit the growth of cariogenic bacteria, particularly oral Streptococci, and prevent it sticking to teeth. Lactoferrin, which is a protein found in breastmilk, kills the bacteria responsible for dental decay (Streptococcus mutans).

Once a child is older than 12 months, the message gets more complicated. Some sources state that continuing to breastfeed after 12 months may increase the risk of dental decay. One systematic review by Tham *et al.* is often cited as making a link between risk of caries and continued breastfeeding (Tham *et al.* 2015).

Tham *et al.* (2015) is a meta-analysis, meaning they are assessing and studying previous research completed by others to try and find the big picture. They did note a relationship between prolonged breastfeeding and dental decay but they describe problems with the way the data was collected (sometimes retrospective interviews) and the fact that variables were not sufficiently controlled.

The authors themselves state that:

Only a few studies included in this review controlled for key confounding factors and this may have resulted in an overestimation of the role of prolonged, frequent and nocturnal breastfeeding in the development of dental caries. Until the dietary and oral hygiene details of these children are controlled for, we cannot be certain whether prolonged, frequent or nocturnal breastfeeding can be principally associated with early childhood caries. (Tham *et al.* 2015)

Another meta-analysis also noted a relationship between prolonged breastfeeding after 24 months and dental caries but described this as being based on low-quality evidence:

> Of the 13,831 papers identified, 627 were screened in duplicate; of these, 139 were included. The highest-level evidence indicated that breastfeeding ≤24 mo does not increase early childhood caries risk but suggested that longer-duration breastfeeding increases risk (low-quality evidence). (Moynihan *et al.* 2019)

Another review, published in 2019, concludes that:

> Breastfeeding until the age of one year is not associated with an increased risk of dental caries, and may even provide protection compared with feeding with formula milk. By contrast, infants who are breastfed beyond the age of 12 months demonstrate an increased risk of caries. However, the results derive from heterogeneous studies that do not always take into account contradictory factors such as eating habits of the mother or infant (feeding during the night, number of meals per day, eating sweet foods, etc.), dental hygiene, or the sociocultural context. (Branger *et al.* 2019)

A newer study has provided more reassurance for families continuing to breastfeed. Devenish *et al.* looked at Australian pre-schoolers in 2020. They studied breastfeeding patterns at three months, six months, 12 months and 24 months. They also looked at the intake of free sugars in the diet. The children had a full dental examination between the ages of two and three to assess the caries rate. They concluded:

> Breastfeeding practices were not associated with early childhood caries. Given the wide-ranging benefits of breastfeeding, and the low prevalence of sustained breastfeeding in this study and Australia in general, recommendations to limit breastfeeding are unwarranted, and breastfeeding should be promoted in line with global

and national recommendations. To reduce the prevalence of early childhood caries, improved efforts are needed to limit foods high in free sugars. (Devenish *et al.* 2020)

It is certainly true that removing other variables is a challenge in this area, as is so often the case when looking at infant nutrition and health. We cannot randomly assign some families to breastfeed, others to not. We cannot ask some families to brush teeth and others to not.

The evidence we have does not convince that breastfeeding to 24 months, or beyond, increases risk of dental caries. Even those who are prepared to state that there is a link will comment on the quality of evidence available and call for more research. If someone claims it is an indisputable fact, we need to consider that they may be basing their opinion more on cultural assumptions about prolonged breastfeeding than the science. If we examine human skeletons from the past, where prolonged breastfeeding and night-time breastfeeding is a given, we see very little signs of decay. It is not unlikely that other variables, such as the increase of sugar in the modern diet, are more of a concern, ahead of what is the biological norm.

> Breastfeeding in itself does not cause caries. That would defy evolution as cave men did not give their children milk from other animals let alone formula. The issue is the modern Western diet whereby we consume very high amounts of sugar. If we restrict sugar intake to a reasonable level (in my opinion and experience that is fruit after meals and very occasional refined sugar products on special occasions) there is no issue with breastfeeding on demand. Offering cows' milk or formula on demand once baby teeth have erupted is a much greater issue as our teeth are not designed to consume them. In a dental study conducted in Tristan da Cunha, the deterioration of oral health on this remote island community was noted in the middle of the 20th century following a change to a diet rich in fermentable

> carbohydrates. This confirms the role of sugar in the aetiology of dental caries.
>
> ~ *(Dentist Richa Sharma)*

The bottom line is that even if a convincing powerful study appeared tomorrow, that had removed all the variables and was flawless in its execution, and it showed that breastfeeding beyond 24 months increased risk of dental decay, this does not mean that extended breastfeeding would not happen. Evidence is beyond dispute that sugars in the diet and fizzy drinks increase risk of tooth decay, and yet adults and children continue to consume these things, because they are making these choices for a multitude of reasons – pleasure, social acceptance, cultural acceptance. The idea that breastfeeding can be 'switched off' and stopped because a professional tells you it should be puts breastfeeding even lower down the list of what is culturally acceptable than fizzy drinks and juice. If a parent says their four-year-old drinks juice or eats biscuits, the chances are the dentist will accept that and explain what else can be done to reduce risk. At most, they may talk about cutting down or offer a sympathetic approach to changing habits. I have yet to hear of a dentist that says, 'Why is your child eating biscuits? There's no value in that.' It goes without saying that it is good practice for a health professional to listen to the families they support, and provide information that supports optimum health of a whole child, not just the bits their training focused on. Does our society value the consumption of cookies ahead of continuing to breastfeed?

What can parents do to reduce risk of dental caries? The list includes drinking a water supply that contains fluoride, no smoking in pregnancy, cleaning teeth properly once teeth appear and regular dental check-ups, minimizing exposure to sugar and understanding that some apparently healthy foods (e.g. dried fruit) may increase risk. Regular snacking in the day could also increase risk. Children should ideally not be offered sugary drinks or juices. Families can be supported to make all these changes without changing breastfeeding patterns. The danger of having conversations which focus on the breastfeeding patterns, and criticize breastfeeding choices, is that parents are more likely to go underground. They may continue to breastfeed without regular dental visits and be less inclined to trust other messages being given. This is true of so many conversations with health professionals: when breastfeeding is devalued or dismissed, an important relationship is damaged and the future health of families may be at risk.

Dr Camila Palma is a paediatric dentist with nearly 20 years' experience. She received her Master's degree from the University of Barcelona, Spain, and she currently has a paediatric dental practice in Lima, Peru, and teaches at the Postgraduate Programme in Paediatric Dentistry at the Peruvian University Cayetano Heredia. She became an IBCLC two years ago.

> I have always been curious about breastfeeding. However, I didn't receive much information about it during my dental education or my specialist training as a paediatric dentist (nor in international congresses). I even recall hearing some of my teacher's prejudices against 'prolonged' breastfeeding but I hadn't learnt about the general and oral benefits of breastfeeding. I used to hear how at-demand breastfeeding was a causative factor for dental caries (and then discovered it's not a cause–effect relationship). My own experience as a mother and the lack of lactation consultants in the dental profession made me venture into the world of lactation. I couldn't be prouder of my decision.
>
> Gaining expertise in breastfeeding has enlarged my professional scope – I not only focus on children's teeth but on their general health, which I never thought I would do. As a paediatric dentist, I have had a good training on oral structures, and as a breastfeeding consultant I have enough experience on breastfeeding issues due to tongue-tie and other oral alterations. Without even realizing, I have become an expert on the diagnosis and treatment of ankyloglossia,

performing frenotomies on a day-to-day basis in newborn babies with breastfeeding problems, which is extremely satisfying.

Solid scientific evidence from systematic reviews shows that children who are exclusively breastfed and who have a longer duration of breastfeeding have a decreased prevalence of malocclusions. This could be explained because: (1) breastfeeding promotes a greater muscular and perioral activity during sucking (compared to bottle-feeding), which in turns stimulates a correct growth and development of all craniofacial structures, and (2) babies who are breastfed have their non-nutritive sucking needs fulfilled and are less prone to use a pacifier or suck their fingers. Non-nutritive sucking habits (pacifier or digit sucking) are significantly associated with malocclusions (especially anterior open bite and posterior crossbite).

The relationship between breastfeeding and dental caries has always been a controversial issue, even between some studies. Most systematic reviews from cohort studies conclude that breastfeeding (beyond the first year), when offered frequently and during the night, is a risk factor for dental caries. However, we have to take into consideration that risk does not mean disease. In no way do these results suggest that breastfeeding be discouraged, but they do support the enhancement of protective strategies for breastfeeding mothers in order to avoid dental caries: mainly using a fluoride toothpaste in adequate amounts before going to bed and avoiding free sugars in the daily diet.

Ending breastfeeding should NEVER be a recommendation to prevent or even to manage dental caries. When mothers decide to continue breastfeeding beyond the first year, dentists should focus on increasing protective factors in order to prevent dental caries and not on discontinuing breastfeeding. Breastfeeding has so many advantages for the overall wellbeing of a child (and mother) that the balance will always be inclined towards maintaining it. The professional who wants to support a change in a patient should have a sensitive and respectful attitude towards his/her lifestyle. Suggesting [to] a parent that their lifestyle is incorrect is not only unfair but also counterproductive to the change we want to promote. Being a parent definitely change[d] my day-to-day practice. I believe I'm a more empathic professional now. As a young graduate student, I remember telling my patient's parents to clean their babies' teeth after offering milk during the night...now I laugh at that recommendation and acknowledge how different theory from practice is! As a mother I now know we all want the best for our children, and we do the best we can with the information we have.

My top three tips for a healthy mouth in children who are breastfed for longer periods of time are:

- To start toothbrushing with a fluoridated toothpaste twice daily from the eruption of the first tooth. It is very important to lift the lip to remove all the milk and food from the upper teeth (the most susceptible to dental decay).

- To avoid free sugars until age two (including packaged juices, cookies, cakes, cereal bars, etc.).

- To visit a paediatric dentist before the baby's first birthday in order to protect its primary teeth with a fluoride varnish and to establish a close relationship with the professional.

I would encourage my fellow dentists to receive training in breastfeeding – there is a whole wide world out there that we do not know much about! And we should! We are the specialists in the oral cavity and its main function is feeding – why aren't we experts on breastfeeding? Moreover, the professional opportunities as a dentist and breastfeeding consultant are amazing: I give lectures around the world, and in my private practice I have so many more children referred by lactation consultants, paediatricians, breastfeeding support groups, nurses, etc.

~ *(Camila Palma)*

We understandably focus on the challenges families face when they talk to health professionals who may lack training in breastfeeding. However, we cannot under-estimate the challenges faced by those who are trained in lactation working alongside colleagues who may not be trained and may not have any personal experience of breastfeeding. There may be even greater challenges if they are working alongside those who do have some personal experience of breastfeeding but either did not reach their feeding goals and are dealing with some trauma, or fed for a short amount of time, and believe anything longer than that is unnecessary.

It is hard to describe the frustration felt when you are up against a system that doesn't 'get' breastfeeding beyond babyhood. You may have to pick up the pieces when parents feel let down. You may have to constantly feel a burden of responsibility as the advocate, pushing for recognition, pushing for more training. It's easy to start to operate in a silo, speaking openly only to those who do share your understanding and avoiding confrontations with those who don't. It can be challenging enough to be an advocate for those breastfeeding small babies: correcting medication errors, facilitating parents staying with their babies, signposting to more specialist care, protecting families from the influence of commercial companies. That can be challenge enough when the evidence around breastfeeding a baby under a few months old is hard for anyone to dispute.

Lucy Upton is a registered dietitian who specializes in paediatrics and is based in the Midlands in England:

> If you are working in a team with other health professionals, you need to be upfront about making sure breastfeeding is seen as a priority. I start by exploring with parents thoughts they have on their journey so far and what are their thoughts about continuing. If it is clear that they want to continue breastfeeding, I like to make everybody aware this is a mum and a family who would like to continue breastfeeding and we need to preserve this. It is stated as a number one aim, not an

afterthought. I ask everyone upfront if they have any concerns about that, in terms of a child's wider medical or social picture if needed, and encourage collaborative discussion. I find people respond positively to this honest but perhaps more proactive and direct approach. We may need to get others involved. What support does mum need? Some mental health support? More specialist support, to support breastfeeding alongside allergy or complex medical diagnosis?

This sounds obvious but it must start with a conversation about breastfeeding with the family. I will admit I have met a breastfeeding family and I have presumed that mum would want to carry on breastfeeding. Then as the case progresses, they may feel 'I've got too much going on' and want to stop and I've had to go back to professionals and say, 'Actually, they don't want to continue breastfeeding.'

The key thing is having a very open forum. If a professional colleague says that they have concerns about breastfeeding, it needs talking about. In the allergy world, it can be frustrating. It can be 'easier' to stop breastfeeding and give formula but 'easier' for who? We should be upskilling everyone so the mum can breastfeed for as long as she wants to. That may mean looking at mum's nutritional requirements too. Parents are often so grateful to feel heard, informed and supported. Regularly, they come to me and say they were expecting to be told to stop breastfeeding. It might have been a worm in their ear telling them that's going to be likely or it's something they've read. They may come with that preconception and that doesn't set you off on the right foot because they're expecting a similar message from you as perhaps other health professionals have told them they need to stop.

Sometimes I am talking to professionals who need further education in breastfeeding. I may not have time to provide support or information, so I'll signpost to other resources, helplines, professionals, e.g. infant feeding advisor (although their time is very limited). You tailor the conversation to the nature of the person that you're talking to and their role. I've worked with paediatricians who were incredibly holistic and incredibly supportive. They often have had personal journeys with breastfeeding themselves and that comes with a background of advocacy, mutual understanding and empathy.

Sometimes doctors will look at the problem in front of them and their brain may skip the significance of breastfeeding and just focus on a solution. If you are open with them and explain its importance, they are usually very supportive. Everything works better when everyone is having open and honest discussion, planning together and communicating together as a team. I appreciate I'm probably 'spoilt' because I work in a big tertiary unit where the whole team is very accessible, and we have more robust training and resources in place. That might be different in district general hospitals/secondary care, or out in the community.

We can signpost to information from UNICEF Baby Friendly or to resources from our infant feeding coordinator and on our intranet. There are always courses available if someone wants to learn more. Having that hands-on experience with families is also really important and that can include shadowing.

It does seem to get harder to advocate for families when they're breastfeeding beyond 12 months. Sometimes there's this rhetoric of 'You have done really well to come this far and there's no need to carry on now because…baby is eating.' There is this heavy weighting towards supporting with the establishing breastfeeding and those first three to six months and then after that it almost feels like it's this pyramid-like dwindling effect. People assume if you've been breastfeeding for 12 months, you don't need support, but even something like reducing feeds isn't as simple as 'just drop a feed'.

Sometimes we are myth-busting, like the myth that breastmilk 'turns to water'. How would that even be possible? Where has that information been heard or sourced from? Even if we don't focus on the nutritional value, we are talking about babies and toddlers going to nursery where they are prone to intercurrent illness. We can't under-estimate the benefit of breastfeeding from the point of view of

> aspects such as immunity. What about human milk oligosaccharides and the ongoing benefit that has for the gut, and overall health?
>
> ~ *(Lucy Upton)*

I appreciate Lucy's comment about needing to start with a conversation with the family. If you are so used to having to advocate for families, it is easy for your enthusiasm to run away with you. Perhaps this is a family that is close to weaning anyway. Perhaps they have no issue with weaning for a medical procedure. We don't want a family to be in a position of feeling as though they are letting us down because our drive to protect natural-term breastfeeding is so strong. We will listen and help parents to explore their feelings and their goals. We will continue to advocate for families and push for resources that help professionals improve their knowledge and look after ourselves in the process.

For parents

Key phrases for nurslings

- 'Big boys can have milk too. I know grown-ups that drink milk and have milk in their tea and coffee.'
- 'Milk helps my brain to grow and protects me against germs.'
- 'Milk eats nasty germs so they don't get into my body.'
- 'Milk helps me relax and go to sleep.'
- 'Milk helps Mummy(/you) to be healthy too.'
- 'Grown-ups do lots of things for comfort. Some of their habits aren't even healthy for them. Mine is.'
- 'What do you do that helps you relax?'

Key phrases for parents (see Chapter 2 for references)

- 'Every 12 months I feed, I have a 4.3% reduction in breast cancer risk.'

- 'A study of 300,000 women found breastfeeding reduces risk of heart disease by 10%.'

- 'An Australian study shows that breastfeeding for longer is associated with positive mental health outcomes into adolescence.'

- 'A study in the Philippines shows longer breastfeeding duration improves social maturity and is associated with better school readiness.'

- 'Continuing to breastfeed reduces my risk of developing type 2 diabetes by 25–47%.'

- 'A 2020 study showed that milk composition from samples at three months and two years were very similar and there was no lost nutritional value. There may even be an increase in fat.'

- 'Some immunological benefits increase in concentration into the second year such as lysozyme, which is a protein that protects against bacteria like E. Coli and salmonella.'

- 'Continuing to breastfeed beyond two years is supported by the World Health Organization, the American Academy of Pediatrics, the American Academy of Family Physicians and every major health organization worldwide.'

- 'The only reason that matters is that we want to continue feeding and it feels right for us. We don't have to give any other reasons.'

Chapter 4

Solid Food Alongside Breastfeeding

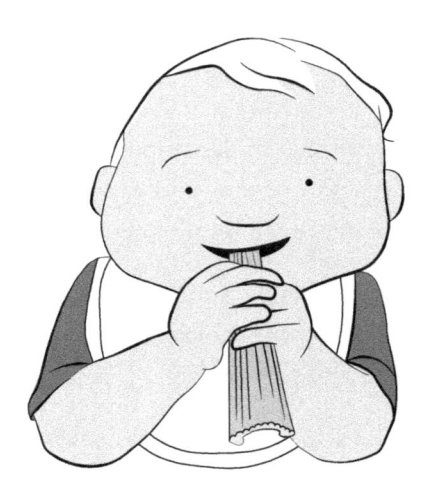

The message to start the introduction of solid foods at around six months has been in place for nearly 20 years. This is the recommendation of the World Health Organization, UNICEF, Health Canada, the UK National Health Service (NHS), the American Academy of Pediatrics, the American Academy of Family Physicians and the Australian National Health and Medical Research Council. Since 2001, the World Health Organization has recommended exclusive breastfeeding for the first six months and then the introduction of solid food alongside breastfeeding. These guidelines were re-affirmed in the 2003 Global Strategy for

Infant and Young Child Feeding from the World Health Organization and UNICEF.

Those of us supporting new families can often be heard to utter the phrase: 'If I had a penny for every time someone told me the guidance was going to change.' However, the reality is that evidence continues to support the introduction of solid food at around six months. The UK government's SACN (Scientific Advisory Committee on Nutrition) published their comprehensive report in 2018, *Feeding in the First Year of Life*, making it clear that 'around six months' remains the recommendation based on the best available science (Public Health England, Scientific Advisory Committee on Nutrition 2018). There have been studies that consider the early introduction of allergens, but in considering these, SACN still affirms that around six months remains the ideal option.

The EAT (Enquiring About Tolerance) study took place from 2008 to 2013 and investigated whether introducing very small amounts of allergens from as early as three months may have a positive effect (Perkin *et al.* 2016). The UK Food Standards Agency (2015) concluded that: 'Overall, food allergy was lower in the group introduced to allergenic foods early but the difference was not statistically significant.'

Professor Amy Brown, in her book *Why Starting Solids Matters*, points out that 'it was challenging to encourage babies this young to consume enough of the target foods' and that 'although these trials show a potential protective impact of early introduction, other studies do not' (Brown 2017, p.36). What is interesting is that the participants in the EAT study had breastfeeding rates that far exceeded usual UK rates, with 96% still breastfeeding at six months compared to the usual national rate of 34% (Renfrew *et al.* 2011). There was still a 50% breastfeeding rate at 12 months, when the best that UK data collection can usually offer is 25% at nine months. If the research team didn't always succeed in supporting parents to feed solid food, perhaps we can ask them what they did around breastfeeding at least.

The reasons to still stick with six months are multiple. This decision is protective of breastfeeding and ensures breastmilk intake doesn't drop.

We know that exclusive breastfeeding to six months is the ideal and makes a contribution to infant and life-long health. Ending exclusive breastfeeding before six months is associated with greater risk of infectious illness. At around six months, the infant gut has matured to the extent that they can better cope with solid food. Plus, at around six months, babies are more likely to be developmentally ready to accept foods and accept a variety of foods and be able to participate and even lead the feeding process.

But what about waiting longer before starting solids? Sometimes when parents are committed to breastfeeding, there can be surprising feelings that arise when it is time for the introduction of solids. You might imagine that it's always a case of holding someone back because the statistics do indicate that it is common for solids to still be introduced before six months. In the UK, in the 2010 infant feeding survey, 75% of parents had introduced solids before their baby was six months old (Renfrew *et al*. 2011). In the USA, more than half introduce solid food before six months (Dallas 2018).

However, in the USA around 13% wait until seven months. Delaying the introduction of solid food does appear to be associated with prolonged exclusive breastfeeding. It is certainly clear that an earlier introduction of solids is associated with formula feeding and a shorter duration of breastfeeding (Barrera *et al*. 2018). We can be confident that exclusive breastfeeding is not associated with a delay in developmental readiness. Those readiness for solid food signs are normally considered to be when a baby is able to sit independently and with a steady head, when they can coordinate their eyes, hands and mouth to be able to move food and bring it to their mouths and when they swallow food, rather than using their tongue to push it back out. Research is clear that breastfeeding aids the development of gross and fine motor skills and does not hinder it (Sacker, Quigley and Kelly 2006). What else might be going on?

I will not be the only lactation consultant who has supported a parent who felt quite tearful at the idea of introducing solids, far from the assumption that new parents are filling their freezers and buying the latest silicone cutlery with glee. Particularly when you have overcome initial breastfeeding challenges and are now exclusively breastfeeding, but perhaps true to anyone who is, there is an enormous satisfaction from knowing you are growing this little person all by yourself. Those fat rolls on the thighs? You did that. The weight chart indicating growth and development? All you. The introduction of solids can sometimes feel more like a loss than a gain. It means a new area to worry about. Parents are bombarded with information about optimum nutrition and overloaded with information that may not always come from ethical sources. They can no longer shield their baby from this world. Solids cost money and may mean less flexibility with travel and daily schedules. It can feel like the end of something as much as the beginning. It has been convenient to breastfeed. Parents can leave the house with very little and their day is their own. They can travel internationally, stay with family, spend a day in the wilderness and they are all their baby needs. Being able to breastfeed has often felt special – baby and parent together protected against outside influence. Plus, starting solids can feel almost like a betrayal of breastfeeding. Breastmilk is a superfood. It may feel disloyal to talk of an insufficiency of micro-nutrients and the importance of adding other sources into the diet. Some parents may also be nervous about the introduction of solids because they fear choking or don't fully understand the difference between choking and gagging.

> Starting solids was actually surprisingly difficult for me. Mateo started eating solids at six months and adjusted to eating three meals a day quite quickly. He enjoyed food! But still also enjoyed several breastfeeds a day. It was actually me who found it difficult. I went from having a portable baby who was reasonably flexible with his schedules and who I could feed whenever or wherever he was hungry, to suddenly having all sorts of restrictions. We had to eat at certain times; he had to eat certain foods so we had to choose cafés

> carefully; and meal preparation, eating and then cleaning up seemed to suddenly take half of my day. It was a huge adjustment for me and caused a period of quite low moods for a while.
>
> ~ (Becky)

All this is to say, if we are supporting breastfeeding parents around the introduction of solids, we need to be sensitive to the possibility of some complex feelings and we must avoid making an assumption that the next stage is 'exciting' and eagerly anticipated. Parents may appreciate empathy and understanding and sometimes practical support such as signposting to a paediatric first aid course.

The iron in breastmilk is uniquely bioavailable but it is sufficient only alongside other sources. For the first six months, this has been the iron reserves laid down in the baby's body. If delayed cord clamping happens at birth, even better. After six months, we are looking at the beginning of other foods. One small study of 30 infants (Pisacane *et al.* 1995) suggested that babies exclusively breastfed until seven months were less likely to have anaemia at 12 months than those who started solids sooner. However, we don't know how their diet developed from seven months, and sources agree that starting to think about alternative sources of iron from six months is likely to be protective for those babies who may take a bit longer to get established with solids. Iron and zinc are micro-nutrients we are particularly concerned about. If solids begin at six months, and it takes some time for swallowing to happen and skills to develop, chances are that quantities will be sufficient by the time iron reserves are running low and additional dietary sources are needed.

Paula Hallam, of tinytotsnutrition.co.uk, is a London-based paediatric dietitian with 20 years of experience working with families:

> If solids are slow to introduce, then the priority is iron-rich foods. I always ask if families are meat-eating families and, if so, to look

> at ways of giving meat to baby. Families sometimes have a bit of a block with meat and giving babies meat and think, 'How on earth am I going to give it?', and babies may struggle with texture which can be quite challenging, so I talk about changing texture with slow-cooking or mincing or puree. Of course there are many other iron-rich options (other than meat) such as iron-fortified cereals, eggs, oily fish, nut butters, beans, lentils, pulses. I talk a lot about prioritizing iron-rich foods. I talk about building a balanced plate for babies and iron-rich foods are the first choice. Other choices come around that (energy-rich and vitamin-rich foods).
>
> ~ *(Paula Hallam)*

Of course, this doesn't mean that breastmilk has lost its value and supplementing breastmilk does not now suggest breastmilk is worthless.

> Sometimes parents are told to stop breastfeeding because breastmilk 'has got no iron in it and requirements are really high', or that baby can get 'everything they need from food now'. I have to correct this regularly, highlighting it isn't now going to be the only source of iron for your baby, but that doesn't negate the importance of breastmilk. Your baby's iron stores are running low and their requirements have gone up. It is an important nutrient, and they need access to iron-rich foods, but breastmilk does still contain some iron (plus it is also very bioavailable), alongside all of the other nutrients, biological factors, etc.
>
> ~ *(Lucy Upton)*

Another reason to start the introduction of solids around six months is about allergy prevention. Some may assume that delaying allergens, or prolonged exclusive breastfeeding, is more protective, but this isn't the case. One study in Japan appeared to find a connection between allergy and prolonged breastfeeding and speculated that the issue may be the delay of the introduction of solid food but more research is needed (Matsumoto *et al.* 2020). A Swedish study published in 2020 concluded: 'Introduction of solids into a child's diet from the age of seven months or later, and maternal history of allergic disease, were both risk factors associated with a higher risk of food allergy or intolerance' (Hicke-Roberts, Wennergren and Hesselmar 2020).

There may also be evidence that suggests delaying the introduction of solids is more associated with later childhood obesity among exclusively breastfed children (Papoutsou *et al.* 2018).

In the face of this evidence, parents may understandably feel under pressure. They are advised to delay until six months but then apparently have a relatively small window in which to 'get things right'.

> There is a lot of conflicting information about what to do – including challenging the phrase and understanding around the 'before one is just for fun', which I challenge regularly. I use this acronym: F is for 'fundamental skill development', U is for 'unique opportunity to learn about food including taste and texture windows' and N is for 'nutrition', including essential nutrients such as iron and zinc. There is a critical window to build the skills and experience, but the word 'critical' might not be right. It gives a sense of urgency and panic for a lot of parents. I'm cautious to put too much pressure on the families, as there is often lots of nerves or worry around complementary feeding. Parents might think babies have got to be eating three meals, plus snacking and managing a full roast dinner already! Lots of people do get misinformation about what to expect from their child when they are starting to eat.
>
> ~ *(Lucy Upton)*

The key message is that the introduction of solids is a gentle one. You may meet an eight-month-old who has still yet to swallow significant amounts but those first taste experiences have been important. Small tastes of iron-rich foods still mean an intake of iron and this is about getting on a road towards the final destination where solid foods will dominate nutritional intake, not pulling out into the fast lane from day one. It's not until 12 months that milk gives less energy than food (First Steps Nutrition Trust 2015, updated 2020). The period of six to seven months is about new experiences for babies but also for parents. Parents are learning to have confidence in their baby's ability to manage food safely. They are introducing a free-running cup with water for the first time, modelling what mealtime looks like and introducing a new world. This is not about cramming in calories but an introduction to a new aspect of family life.

Baby-led weaning is a method of introducing solid food that is commonly associated with breastfeeding. It involves the child self-feeding from the beginning and food staying in its natural state as far as is sensible. Rather than their meal of peas, lentils and chicken consisting of a mush of these ingredients combined into a uniform colour, they stay recognizable. In front of them will be pieces of cooked chicken, or even a chicken drumstick they can gnaw on, perhaps a patty made from lentils and peas they can practise their pincer grip on. Despite its name, baby-led weaning does not refer to weaning from the breast but a more traditional use of the term that meant introducing other foods. For breastfeeding parents, the method often feels like a natural extension of breastfeeding. Babies are in charge, just as they are at the breast. Quantities are not measured in millilitres or oz but in what feels sensible. Baby-led weaning encourages a baby to listen to its own appetite, to explore and to quickly become part of normal family mealtime. Barring the usual restrictions such as honey before 12 months, choking hazards and high levels of salt, the baby eats normal family foods. It may take some time for quantities to develop. In the early days, the experience of food is about colour and texture and playful exploration. There is no parent-led spooning of amounts or a belief that a jar or bowl should be emptied. The rate of progress will also be led by the baby and it may take them some time before they are eating three full meals a day, as evidence in the nappy will show.

Stacey Zimmels is the owner of Feed Eat Speak (a feeding and speech therapy service for infants and children), and a speech and language therapist and IBCLC who specializes in paediatric feeding and swallowing:

> There is no clear time frame regarding when to progress from [one to two to three] meals per day when introducing solids. However, many 'weaning experts' in their books and on social media promote the idea that a baby could be on three meals a day by seven months of age. For breastfeeding mothers who follow this advice the consequence is very likely that the breastfed infant will significantly reduce milk volumes, in order to accommodate solid foods.
>
> ~ (Stacey Zimmels)

Anxiety around introducing lumpier food or new foods may mean a baby is given a more limited range of foods for longer, so parental confidence is key. Parents appreciate understanding that food rejection is very normal and a baby may need to be offered a food more than ten times before it is accepted. If a baby is uninterested in solids, we never force a mouthful, but they may respond well to some mashed food on a spoon. Other babies are self-feeding pros and baby-led weaning and breastfeeding often feel like natural partners. As breastfed babies, they have been in charge. Now with baby-led weaning, where the child is offered a range of finger foods and encouraged to self-select and self-feed, that independence continues. Breastfed babies are more likely to be adventurous with trying new foods, and one theory is this is because they are used to the varying tastes of breastmilk. Research suggests: 'it would seem that both breastfeeding and the timely introduction of a variety of tastes and food textures would best predict acceptance and subsequent inclusion of a wide range of foods, especially fruit and vegetables, within the child's diet' (Harris and Coulthard 2016).

Parents sometimes feel confused about how breastfeeding continues alongside solid food. In the bottle-feeding world, we hear talk of 'dropping' feeds. How does this translate to breastfeeding?

> We don't expect a big decrease in milk intake in the first few months, it is a very gradual decrease in milk and increase in solids from six months of age. We might encourage parents to think 'milk first' initially but there aren't definite rules. Some babies will take to solids and some will need a bit of a nudge, especially if they love the boob and don't seem to really want anything else. They might need a bit of encouragement. Initially, we wouldn't want milk volume to decrease. Introducing solids is about tastes, and introducing tastes and milk stays about the same in the early days of weaning. I think sometimes people have a picture in their mind, and this might sometimes come from conversations with a medical professional (perhaps in allergy prevention), that foods have to be introduced quickly, even aggressively. This isn't the case. They might have expectations that quickly babies will be on just a couple of milk feeds. Parents might feel like a failure if they haven't managed to introduce all these foods.
>
> It's rare to need to encourage a family to reduce breastfeeding as usually it's more about scheduling and trying to minimize a 'boob monster' grazing on the breast and snacking throughout the day. Of course, breastmilk is still nutritious. Sometimes I meet families who have been told by doctors that breastmilk stops being nutritious after one year of age, but that's not the case. Introducing a routine to reduce constant time on the breast and creating some space for food might be useful.
>
> ~ *(Paula Hallam)*

Breastfeeding parents rarely need to make any conscious decisions around milk intake. There is a natural adjustment as exposure to solids gradually increases and dependence on milk shifts. A nursling will handle their own intake. It's only if we get to eight to ten months, and solids intake hasn't increased, that we might do some nudging. This might mean no longer thinking 'milk first' and offering solids first. Paula Hallam sometimes suggests that parents shift around the first feed of the day:

> If a baby isn't showing much interest in solids at around nine or ten months, what can work is switch in the morning. Rather than doing a big milk feed on wake-up, they might try food first and then breastfeed afterwards.
>
> ~ *(Paula Hallam)*

It isn't always as straightforward as switching milk and solids to encourage more solids intake. Care needs to be individualized.

> When it comes to introducing solids there is no set time in which a baby 'should' progress with their eating. Like with all aspects of infant feeding it is best if the progression is baby led and responsive. Begin by introducing tastes/a single meal at the family table, and depending on how your baby takes to this then you would introduce a second meal. Breastfeeds can be offered before solids so that baby comes to the table in a state where they are going to be able to learn the skills of eating and not too hungry (or tired for that matter).
>
> ~ *(Stacey Zimmels)*

What about if more months go by and there are still concerns? It can be tempting for a parent to blame themselves, but of course, there are professionals who are available for support.

Again, support will be individualized.

> I saw a 12-month-old who wasn't eating any solids beyond a few spoons of prune puree with a lot of distractions. Her mother was returning to work (at home) and in anticipation had reduced daytime feeds in order to 'help' get her eating. She was feeding her first thing in the morning and then not again until after lunch. It hadn't worked and she was very reluctant to even sit in the highchair at lunchtime. In our first consultation I suggested reintroducing a mid-morning and mid-afternoon feed so that she was not too hungry at lunchtime. When I reviewed her after a month, her mother reported that by changing the timings of milk feeds she was much happier, she was willing to sit in the highchair for lunch and dinner and was exploring and beginning to taste some finger foods.
>
> ~ *(Stacey Zimmels)*

If a child is 14 or 15 months and eating food hasn't taken off, I look at supporting the whole family. I usually get them to write down their whole routine and have a wider conversation about expectations. I think sometimes that helps take the pressure off because usually at this point mothers, parents or wider family can start to feel to blame. They think, 'Is it because I've continued breastfeeding?' I certainly see that worry a lot. People think, 'Is this my fault?' I ask about all of the routine: what's their sleep like, what is their mealtime routine? I usually ask for a video of a mealtime so I can see what the child is doing, how they are eating, what mealtimes are like and what's the communication or interactions like between child and parent. How is the response when we start to get to that toddler age where they have those tantrums and those developmental changes? If breastfeeding is being used for comfort, that's obviously fine but it can be helpful to explore other factors to support comfort and regulation too. Sometimes parents get stuck with offering a limited range of food, sometimes sticking with giving foods their child will eat. Sometimes that can be puree – often sweet! Sometimes that can be the same sort of foods on repeat. I look at family mealtime and encourage eating with others/the family regularly and having that as a crucial part of their routine. I will probably be looking to establish parental understanding around what you would expect your normal toddler eating routine to look like. Toddlers may be getting crabby at mealtimes and not want to sit as long at the table, or parents may have disproportionate expectations of a mealtime both with what and how much a toddler will eat. In one recent video, which I was able to share with parents, I could see a baby getting tiresome of mealtime at ten minutes – this was the time to end the mealtime; however, the mealtime persisted for 35 minutes, by which point the child was very upset and frustrated!

I also help parents to understand how a baby's growth is changing, that it is slowing down and that means that their energy requirements drop at 12 months. So many people think, 'Bigger child therefore must mean bigger portions.' You can see how that assumption develops. It makes logical sense, but in the 12 months between 12 months and 24 months, there's about 20% drop in energy requirements. Of course, there might be a small proportion of those 14- and 15-month-olds who actually have developmental issues, so if I have got more global concerns regarding their development, I will get a broader team involved.

~ *(Lucy Upton)*

Marina Ferrari is an IBCLC and also has a background in nutrition. She emphasizes:

Solid Food Alongside Breastfeeding

> In situations where breastfeeding is taking too much space in baby's diet because of non-nutritional needs, restricting breastfeeding is not the answer. Actually, reducing breastfeeding could impact baby's nutrition even more. Breastfeeding reduction might be the consequence of the professional approach, but shouldn't be the recommendation.
>
> ~ (Marina Ferrari)

She also points out the irony that the myths surrounding breastfeeding beyond six months contain two diametrically opposed concepts: that breastmilk loses its nutritional value AND if you aren't cautious too much breastmilk may mean a child doesn't increase their intake of solids appropriately. Truthfully, the process of introducing solid food in addition to breastfeeding is a straightforward one for the vast majority of children. Milk continues to be the main source of energy and nutrients for quite some time. The opportunity of solids begins and a transition gradually occurs where solid food becomes increasingly important and more about meeting the needs of hunger and not just about giving an experience.

If the intake of solids is very slow to develop, families are sometimes told to cut back on breastfeeding. However, this isn't a course of action supported by many specialists in this area.

> Eating is a skill which needs to be learnt. Whilst having an appropriate appetite is an important driver for eating it is not the only thing that is required for an infant/child to eat. Stopping or cutting breastfeeds is not necessarily a solution to supporting eating. If a baby doesn't have the skills to eat or there is something else going on which is holding up their progress with eating then it still won't help them. Removing a baby's only source of nutrition in an attempt to get them eating when they haven't yet shown you they can do it can be harmful and can result

> in weight loss. In addition, breastfeeding is not just providing an infant with nutrition; intervening drastically with reduction of breastfeeding will impact their source of comfort, connection, sleep and can also result in a hungry baby.
>
> ~ (Stacey Zimmels)

The reduction of breastfeeding may be a consequence of professional support but a call to reduce breastfeeding is not an entire professional approach in itself. A reduction or re-patterning of breastfeeding may occur as approaches to increase the intake of solid food are successful.

In rare cases, a reluctance to eat solid food may be associated with an allergy. If a baby was diagnosed as having an allergy before solids, the parent is also likely to be anxious. During breastfeeding, they had complete control over intake. They may have undertaken an elimination diet but it became something that they grew accustomed to and even a slip-up will mean exposure to a small quantity. There is 100,000 times less cows' milk protein conveyed through breastmilk than from direct exposure to cows' milk as a drink (Jones 2019). It can be tempting to continue the cocoon of breastfeeding, but as we've seen there is evidence that delaying solids may increase rather than reduce allergy risk. It is also possible that introducing solids brings the first signs of an allergic reaction previously not noted during breastfeeding.

> I was really excited to start J on solids at exactly six months! However, this excitement quickly fizzled out as it became apparent how messy and time-consuming the process was! We did a combination of purees and baby-led weaning. Again looking back this isn't something I plan on doing with O – I'll just do baby-led weaning as will lack the time or energy to be making lots of purees! J took to solids pretty well – our only real issue was the cows' milk protein allergy which only became evident on starting solids (she never reacted to dairy via

> breastmilk). Her reactions were hives, vomiting and distress within five minutes of eating dairy. This was obviously worrying, but again in retrospect I feel that some positives have come out of this experience as it triggered an interest in allergies for me. It made starting childcare and being around other children eating stressful as most people have very limited awareness of allergies, e.g. not reading labels properly or understanding that even a small amount can cause a reaction. She outgrew her allergy at around 20 months.
>
> ~ *(Naomi)*

Does a breastfeeding older child ever need cows' milk? Technically no one needs to drink cows' milk, of course. There has been a lot of effort over many decades focused on convincing parents that milk has magical properties, but truthfully, it contains nothing that cannot be found elsewhere. It's not unusual for an older nursling to wean from breastfeeding and show no interest in drinking cows' milk at all. That can be a time when some parents worry. It may even prevent them from weaning from breastfeeding when that is something that they want to do.

> There is sometimes a message that babies over 12 months need cows' milk. If a baby is breastfeeding three or four times, cows' milk isn't needed. Even if they are feeding just twice a day, they don't need cows' milk if they are eating dairy and things like yoghurt, cheese, etc. I sometimes say to parents that calcium requirements over one year [old] are smaller than you might think, less than in the first year. You don't have to introduce cows' milk as an actual drink. When an older child does wean and doesn't want to drink cows' milk, that's not a problem. Cows' milk itself is not essential. The nutrients in it are essential. As long as a child is getting enough calcium, iodine, protein and energy from other foods, they don't need to drink cows' milk. From one to three years, the calcium requirement is 350mg. From

four years, it goes up a little bit, progressively more. If a family... doesn't want to include dairy in their diet [they] might use soya, soya products and other non-dairy sources of calcium. They may need to access support to get further information. It's perfectly possible for a child to grow up never having had cows' milk.

~ *(Paula Hallam)*

Chapter 5

Breastfeeding and Sleep

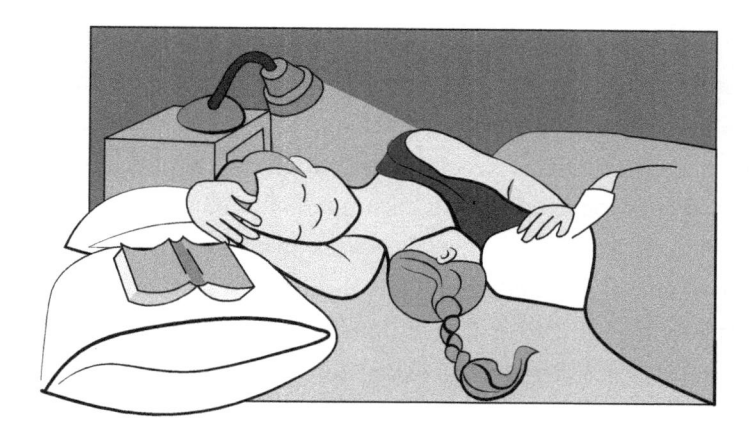

What is normal for a young child in terms of sleeping patterns? There is a lot of normal. In a large 2014 Australian study, parents recorded sleeping and napping patterns in their children aged zero to nine years. They noted 'huge variation at all ages in sleep duration, sleep onset time and, especially, wake time in this normal population' (Price *et al.* 2014). In one 2010 study, more than a quarter of 12-month-olds were not sleeping through from 10 pm to 6 am. Researchers found 13% were not sleeping continuously from midnight to 5 am (Henderson *et al.* 2010). In one 2017 study of 2800 children, about 50% of the two-year-old children woke one or two times per night (Kocevska *et al.* 2017).

Waking to breastfeed does not automatically mean reduced sleep quality for parents. Research has shown that new parents who are exclusively breastfeeding get more sleep (contrary to some assumptions). At one month, 'Women who breastfed exclusively averaged 30 minutes more nocturnal sleep than women who used formula at night' (Doan *et al.* 2014). It seems that this effect may continue beyond the initial post-partum period. A 2013 study looking at parents of infants aged zero to 12 months found that parental sleep was improved when families were exclusively breastfeeding (Kendall-Tackett, Cong and Hale 2013).

It does appear that when a child is continuing to breastfeed and also to bedshare, they may wake more frequently (Elias *et al.* 1986). Our idea of a normal toddler sleeping pattern is likely to be different in societies where bedsharing continues to be the norm. A child that is rousing may also be going back to sleep quickly. They will be rousing between sleep cycles rather than experiencing 'broken' sleep, and parents who have sleep cycles that are in sync with their nurslings may also be well rested. What is our biological norm? In how much of human history have young children been sleeping in separate spaces away from parents and having a human milk diet ended after a few months? In fact, our norm may be 'breastsleeping'. Anthropologists James McKenna and Lee Gettler use this term to describe a natural sleep state for a young child:

> for breastfeeding mothers, the decision to bedshare proves often to be an unexpected 'no brainer' explaining why, perhaps, a quiet but seismic shift towards adopting bedsharing in Western cultures... is occurring as breastfeeding re-establishes itself in many Western countries as the cultural norm. (McKenna and Gettler 2016)

Continuing to wake past 12 months as a nursling is not unusual. IBCLC Meg Nagle polled more than 8000 parents and found 66% of nurslings over 24 months fed between one and three times overnight. She found 12% were feeding four to six times. Nagle says, 'They do not have sleep problems. These are breastfed kids who are continuing to do what babies and young children have always done since...forever! They are waking at night to find some comfort through breastfeeding' (Nagle 2021).

As Nagle points out, there may be times a child is frequently waking because something isn't quite right. They may be uncomfortable or have a condition that requires medical assistance, but if they wake calmly, feed happily, go back to sleep peacefully, that can be considered normal and not abnormal.

Some parents hear about what is normal and commonly experienced by other breastfeeding families and feel a huge sense of relief. They didn't feel like anything HAD to change. They just had a creeping feeling that this wasn't how things were supposed to be. The rest of the world seemed to be sleeping through, sleeping in separate spaces, sleeping without contact between child and parent. Were they supposed to be doing something different? Were they somehow failing their child by not moving things forward? Truthfully, bedsharing and child/parent contact at night is normal in most places but just not always talked about. In Japan, bedsharing is seen as the norm but the rates are not significantly higher than in the USA (McKenna 2007). Once parents appreciate that breastfeeding an older child through the night continues to be normal, they can often relax. As Meg Nagle says:

> I promise you, your child WILL eventually fall asleep on their own and sleep in their own bed. Believe me…my 14-year-old who spent the first few years of his life breastfeeding cuddled up next to me, would cringe at the thought of me cuddling him to sleep now! They do grow up. In the meantime? Cuddle them. You simply cannot breastfeed your child too often or cuddle them too much. (Nagle 2021)

However, that sense of relief and acceptance isn't true for everyone. Some were hoping this wasn't normal and it was either temporary or fixable. They may seek the support of a sleep professional. Lyndsey Hookway has a background as a paediatric nurse, health visitor and IBCLC. She writes and speaks on several aspects of caring for babies and children and developed the holistic sleep coaching programme which is an internationally renowned family-centred approach to sleep support.

Her books include: *Still Awake: Responsive Sleep Tools for Toddlers to Tweens* (2021), *Let's Talk About Your New Family's Sleep* (2020) and *Holistic Sleep Coaching: Gentle Alternatives to Sleep Training for Health and Childcare Professionals* (2018).

I asked Lyndsey some questions.

Q. Supporting parents with sleep sometimes means talking about what's normal. What are you often normalizing?
Every family has their own sleep situation, challenges and questions. That said, there are a number of recurring themes that come up in relation to sleep:

1) the amount of sleep a child needs

2) nap confusion

3) night feeds.

It's really important to have a realistic reference point for average sleep needs. Many people think that their child is sleep deprived because their child might not sleep as long as someone else's baby sleeps. Children's sleep falls within a range, and most of the time, children are getting plenty of sleep, albeit not in a convenient way. It is normal for children to experience fragmented sleep. The important distinction is the difference between sleep fragmentation, and sleep deprivation. Infant and young toddler sleep is likely to lead to adult sleep deprivation, because it is normal for them to need parental help to fall back to sleep between sleep cycles, but prompt, responsive care means that these brief awakenings are inconsequential for children, though disruptive for parents. It's important to remember that all of us wake briefly between sleep cycles in the night – this does not mean we are sleep deprived. It's common for parents to believe that their child needs more sleep than they are actually getting. Understanding what is normal is vital, because there is only so much sleep a child can achieve in 24 hours. Putting them to bed too early, for example, may lead to more sleep fragmentation at night, due to insufficient sleep pressure.

Naps are another major area of confusion that often needs some normalizing. Parents may be concerned that their baby only takes short naps, only ever naps while being held or carried, or fed to sleep, or they may be bothered about the timing of naps. It's a myth that more daytime sleep always leads to more night-time sleep – because, again, there is only so much sleep that a child can achieve in 24 hours. Having really long naps may in fact be the cause of fragmented nights. It is also normal for infants and young toddlers to prefer to sleep in close proximity to their parent. This is only a problem if it is a problem for the parent.

The other common area that often needs some normalizing is night feeds – which continue to be normal into the second year and beyond. A more difficult conversation is when night waking is really frequent, or becoming unsustainable. People might reach out and say that they know their ten- or 15-month-old baby is going to wake up at night and need to be comforted, and that's fine. They just don't think their baby needs to feed every hour. This can be really hard, especially if parents have gone back to work at this point. Again, there are plenty of ways to make gentle, respectful changes to sleep without using a non-responsive approach.

Q. What do you sometimes suggest if parents are struggling with frequent waking?
There are many small hacks and improvements that can be made. It's not within the scope of a small section in a book to describe all of these, but one option is to try to relax about sleep. It's easy for sleep to become an obsession that can take over the day. I've often found that when everybody calms down about sleep, it spontaneously gets a little bit better. Furthermore, a parent who is less stressed may feel less fatigued, and will experience better quality sleep.

If a child is waking hourly this can be really tough. While it may be as simple as a child just briefly awakening after each sleep cycle, this can get pretty exhausting after a while. If children are waking very frequently, and especially if they are fatigued in the daytime, it is worth ruling out a medical cause for night waking. This may include mouth-breathing, sleep disordered breathing, a feeding problem, weight problem, ear infection or another condition.

Once other issues have been ruled out, what sometimes helps with frequent waking is to increase sleep pressure by having a later bedtime, less daytime sleep, or a longer chunk of awake time before bed. This often consolidates sleep. This simple intervention is a good place to start because this involves no overnight sleep modification at all, it just allows their sleep biology and their body rhythm to do a little bit of the legwork.

Q. Is it a concern if a nursling uses the breast to help them get to sleep?

Feeding to sleep is normal, common and, like so many other sleep and parenting behaviours, is only a problem if it is becoming problematic for a parent. Lots of people ask if babies can develop a habit of feeding back to sleep. I think it is fair to say that babies can develop a preference for how they want to be supported or parented back to sleep. If you try and offer them another way of going back to sleep, then they may object – loudly. Sending in another parent sometimes works, or sometimes this makes babies really angry and upset.

One of my favourite strategies for helping babies get used to other ways of being parented back to sleep is habit-stacking. It's not reasonable to think that you can just switch out feeding to sleep or holding to sleep and think that a baby is going to find that immediately soothing. Habit-stacking is based on behaviour change psychology and involves overlapping some new, and more sustainable, strategies that help ease a child away from their favourite one, while still maintaining responsiveness. The parent gradually peels away the layers of sleep support that they find difficult, leaving the more sustainable ones. It enables the baby to begin to associate the process of being really loved and nurtured and calmed to sleep with something else other than feeding. It's not quick and it requires some patience, but this is usually a very gentle option.

With older children, it often helps to set some boundaries in the daytime first. Allowing children to come up against those limits and boundaries in the daytime is easier. It's really difficult for kids to learn hard things at hard times of the day. I often suggest doing hard things at easy times. I also talk about the need for parents to not always distract their child from their big feelings about those boundaries. Sometimes people say no but try to distract by offering a cracker or new activity. However, it's important to allow a child to feel what they feel, with the emotional support from a parent.

Q. Parents are often given information about sleep training methods. Why is that still so common?
One of the main problems is that the research we currently have on sleep training appears to suggest that there is no long-term harm of leaving infants to cry. Unfortunately, the research has been heavily criticized by many for the small sample sizes, large drop-out rates, methodological flaws, lack of diversity and relatively short follow-up times. Ultimately the best we can say at the moment is that there is no solid evidence of harm per se, but there is also no definitive proof of safety. Furthermore, the other big issue is that leaving a child to cry, for many parents, just feels wrong. Most parents would choose another option if they knew about it.

I can see the appeal of sleep training methods. The main behavioural sleep training methods – gradual retreat, pick up, put down, controlled crying and full extinction – are easy and quick to describe. Most of the gentler strategies take a lot more time to explain, understand and require more time investment. They also require more understanding of sleep biology.

> A lot of the more gentle-minded health visitors, of whom there are thousands, will naturally lean towards evidence-based organizations like Basis (Baby Sleep Information Source). These organizations are wonderful for normalizing sleep and providing research on bedsharing. The only problem is that hearing that something is normal may not be enough to help the parent on the end of the phone to the duty health visitors saying, 'I'm literally about to walk out, I feel so sleep deprived and deranged because of tiredness.' There is a problem because health professional training doesn't fully meet the needs of either the service providers or the service users. If a parent is only told about sleep training techniques, then they may choose to do nothing. If a parent is only told that their child is normal – they may turn to sleep training in desperation. Both of these outcomes are disempowering and they won't have addressed the problems the parent had when they made that call. We need better, more comprehensive training for health professionals that goes beyond the two extremes of either normalizing everything, or recommending sleep training.

At the risk of sounding like a broken record, there is not one way that all families breastfeeding older children approach sleep. Some families will bedshare and a nursling will have unrestricted access to the breast throughout the night. This may be a situation that a family cherishes. It may be a situation that a family actively encourages. This may be a family where the baby has never been allocated a separate sleep space and there is no equivalent to a cot even in the house. They may be working parents who encourage unrestricted breastfeeding at night to prevent the need for milk to be provided in the day. However, a different family with the exact same scenario may feel as though they are a family in crisis and in desperate need of support. One parent may be happy, the other may not be. Both parents may be struggling. There is enormous variation in what is happening and how parents feel about it.

I night weaned J at a fairly early age (14 months) because I couldn't see any other way of getting more sleep. She was waking up to five times per night and sometimes awake for two hours at a time. I was back at work and beyond exhausted. I night weaned her in a very harsh manner, which I really regret and I hope she doesn't remember it. I couldn't see any other way out, but I plan to do things very differently with O.

~ *(Naomi)*

I don't think night-time parenting is ever going to be easy. It's exhausting and draining, but I was well aware from lots of research I had read that breastfeeding doesn't necessarily increase the frequency of night-time wake-ups. Meaning a night weaned child may still wake often, but no longer has a guaranteed way to settle them back to sleep!

~ *(Millie)*

At night she still feeds a lot. She will start off asleep in her bed but wakes up in the night and that's when she comes to my bed and we bedshare. My husband changes bed as well. Lots of couples we know aren't so flexible, but for us it means we can all get more sleep and no one is distressed trying to keep an upset toddler in her bed, when she wants to be with me. Plus we all actually enjoy it!

We always feed from my left breast during the night and I can definitely tell that one produces more milk than the right. If I start a daytime feed off with the right breast, Olive will often want to switch to the left after a few minutes saying 'more'.

~ *(Nikki)*

My daughter woke a lot during the nights, and feeding her back to sleep whilst bedsharing was the easiest way for all of us so we could all get the most sleep. With my son (nearly 11 months), we bedshare, and

> feeding to sleep is also so much easier than having to carry to sleep. It's also the easiest way to comfort any upset, be it an illness or teething, etc. I don't know what I would do without my boob 'magic'…
>
> ~ (Eve)
>
> I fed Ralphie throughout the night until about 13 months when my body had had enough. I was so tired from co-sleeping and constant feeding and I just needed to get a proper sleep. We then put him in his own room and stopped feeding at night. It was glorious!
>
> ~ (Anna)
>
> My child is almost four and likes to feed to sleep with me – she has a bath and a story and then I feed her – I love this part of the day as I relax with her and ask her if she wants to tell me anything before I say the same thing I've said every night for years and she drifts off. Sometimes she de-latches before she is asleep and will roll over and go to sleep whilst I look at my phone or read and then get up and go downstairs. We co-sleep, and over the last few months I've said I can't keep doing night feeds overnight and have asked her to have water or a cuddle and she's adapted to that now.
>
> ~ (Nat)

One breastfeeding three-year-old may sleep from 7 pm to 7 am without a murmur, another may wake for a breastfeed every 60 to 90 minutes. Is it the breastfeeding that is the relevant variable here? Could it be a relationship to breastfeeding? When breastfeeding has a wider significance for child and maternal health, the notion that ending breastfeeding should be an automatic response to a sleep issue that may or may not be breastfeeding-related seems strange. Yet it is familiar to hear a story where a family are struggling with sleep and the concept of stopping breastfeeding is the only solution offered. It may be accompanied by a comment that a child is 'too attached' or 'needs more independence'. What is often extremely painful is when breastfeeding is ended through desperation but sleep issues continue and problems are unresolved. The family has lost a way to deliver sedatives into their child regularly through the night on top of dealing with sleep difficulties. What is ideal is a full exploration of all the factors that may be at play before quick decisions are made. This could be with the support of someone knowledgeable about normal breastfeeding patterns and sleep in a child of the right age.

Night weaning is an option for many parents who feel they have reached the end of their limits and it can help and does not mean an end to breastfeeding overall. Sometimes meeting the nursling's requests to feed continuously through the night no longer feels compatible with the family's best interest. As Dr Jay Gordon describes:

> I really don't like listening to babies cry. I actually hate listening to babies cry. Unlike them, though, we adults can truly understand the implications of lack of sleep for a family of three, four or more people. Sleep patterns sometimes have to be changed. The incredible safety and reassurance the family bed has provided, and continues to provide, supplies the best context and location for these changes. (Gordon 2020)

It is important to begin with some reflection. What are the goals here? If there is an assumption that night weaning means a child who no longer wakes at night, that is not something that can be guaranteed. If a parent is feeling over-stretched, what other areas of their life can they make changes in? This may not be easiest. Are there other barriers to their child sleeping well? Could it be that napping in the day needs adjusting and a child is under-tired? Could they be ready for a different sleep environment with more room? Could something else be causing issues such as allergy, environmental noise and use of light in the sleeping space?

If a parent has reflected and feels night weaning is something that they want to try, this may bring some upset. However, this doesn't mean that crying is the aim nor that the only way to night wean is by a harsh approach devoid of empathy. It is possible to night wean and for a parent to still be true to their parenting instincts. Their child is going to need their help. They are being asked to fall asleep in a new way and that takes re-learning a skill and saying goodbye to a much-loved habit.

Parents may already be familiar with the 'Pantley pull-off' from *The No-Cry Sleep Solution for Toddlers and Pre-Schoolers* by Elizabeth Pantley (2005). A nursling begins to feed as normal, but rather than continuing until they are in a deep sleep, they are gently detached when they are merely sleepy. They may protest and seek the breast again. A parent may re-attach them but still break off the feed before deep sleep happens. Parents may also bring in other tools that start to be associated with sleep time. It might be a story perhaps, a way of patting or a cuddly toy. With older children, they may be able to talk about the change that is going to happen in the family routine. They may understand that breastfeeding only happens when the sun comes up. This concept is captured in the book *Nursies When the Sun Shines*, which could be read to a child (Havener 2013). Some parents make their own book using family photos and familiar phrases.

A family that is choosing to night wean may still choose to have a bedtime feed and even allow a nursling to fall asleep at the breast last thing at night, but when a waking in the middle of the night happens, new strategies come into play. Some older children can appreciate the connection that it is now night-time and 'milkies are asleep' or 'it's cuddling time'. Some families use a clock designed for a young child, where a bunny's ears pop up when it's morning or a colour on the clock changes when it's time for milk again. I did however once hear a story of a rabbit clock that suffered considerably when a nursling used all their ingenuity to try and get the ears to pop up in the dead of night. A parent may use key phrases softly spoken. They may pat gently or lie nearby. They may sit in a chair and make it known they are there and they are not alone. They may place a mattress on the floor so non-breastfeeding cuddles can be an option and a family that uses a cot has an option other than 'in the cot' or 'in the chair where breastfeeding historically happens'. In some families where the child has their own room, a chair may gradually move towards the door (assuming the child is sleeping in a different room) and one day even be outside the door. Families will find strategies that work for them that make it clear that just because milk is being removed, the feeling that someone is there to support you has not been. Sometimes the tiniest changes can make a difference. Wearing different clothing that means the breast is less accessible can mean there is enough of a barrier that a half-asleep nursling thinks 'forget it' and falls back to sleep with a little hand on the pyjama buttons.

Embarking on a process of night weaning requires commitment. It needs parents who are absolutely confident this is the approach they want to take as it is not going to be easy. There may be tears and protests, and if a parent is unsure, it is going to be challenging to create that consistent and solid environment. Having said that, every parent has the right to change their mind and decide the process of night weaning is not for them but that then perhaps means a break from attempting rather than re-starting 72 hours later. Starting a process of night weaning also requires physical energy. Many families don't do it as what they are currently tolerating (often regular feeding and co-sleeping) does mean that everyone is getting sleep. They may be unhappy with the current patterns and struggling but still the concept of summoning the energy to night wean is too much. Not letting a nursling fall asleep on the breast means that the parent has to stay awake too, when often they may latch a child back on and fall asleep themselves. Saying no and offering alternative methods of comfort may mean angry protesting that lasts an hour. The concept of fitting that into their lives can feel too much.

When a family makes a choice to embark on night weaning it requires preparation. This is a time to call in the troops. With a two-parent household, one may be assigned a day of gentle rest and napping to be able to take the lead when night comes. The parent who has taken the lead overnight gets the chance to lie in the next day. It may be a time to call in other family members or friends for an early morning visit and a trip to the park while parents go back to bed. It's a time for ordering food in and minimizing other stresses. Some families take days off work and use a family holiday for night weaning. Others start on a Friday night. Night weaning should not feel like a battle. This is not parents versus nursing. This is about team work. The day before a first attempt at night weaning may be a day to offer the breast even more than is normal. It's a day for cuddles and togetherness. The day after a night of weaning attempts is also a day for rewards and connection.

Some parents prefer to start with blocks of time when they won't be feeding at night but then accept feeding at other times. Dr Jay Gordon has written a plan for families who wish to night wean and sleep in a family bed. He advocates selecting a key seven hours and focusing on those (Gordon 2020). He describes how a baby with a 'well-built' personality will be able to accommodate a change of rules for this time. For the first three nights, a nursling could be fed upon waking but they must be put back down awake. That might mean a shorter feed. They are not able to fall asleep while feeding. Parents may expect some protest:

> Now, he will tell you that he is angry and intensely dislikes this new routine. I believe him. He will also try to tell you that he's scared. I believe he's angry, but a baby who's had hundreds of nights in a row of cuddling is not scared of falling asleep with your hand on his back and your voice in his ear. Angry, yes. Scared, no, not really. (Gordon 2020)

The nursling will be settled to sleep in a different way. That might be patting or comforting with a cuddle. Feeding cannot happen again until they have slept and re-awakened. Then the next three nights, when waking happens in that seven-hour block, Dr Gordon suggests feeding is not on offer. Again, you might cuddle and do whatever else helps your nursling to settle but they will fall back asleep without the breast. It might take them 15 minutes or an hour. The next four nights, slightly downshift on the method of comfort, so not picking up but a pat and a soothing voice. Dr Gordon describes how the process ends:

> After these first ten nights, continue to cuddle and feed to sleep if you like and he wants to, but do nothing when he wakes up except to touch a little and talk to him briefly. This may continue for another three or four nights but occasionally keeps going for another week or more. Then...it stops. He has learned that he is just as well-loved, gets virtually everything he needs and wants all day, but must give seven hours per night back to his parents and family. (Gordon 2020)

The process works because the love cup is being filled, rather than it being a story of loss and deprivation. Not everyone would be comfortable with a prescriptive plan to structure certain behaviours around a set number of nights. It may be that a family prefers to stay in one phase for longer than Dr Gordon outlines or adapt according to what feels appropriate, but it can be useful to have an idea of a structure. It can also be useful to have 'permission' to make changes to a family's approach to sleep and permission to be able to prioritize the parent's needs. A parent who has continued breastfeeding and was anticipating child-led weaning, perhaps alongside attachment parenting, can have feelings of guilt when they consider changing night-time behaviour. As is often the case with any aspect of parenting an older breastfeeding child, parents can struggle with the idea that they are able to focus on their own needs. It is important to remind them that addressing a sleep situation that doesn't work for them may mean that the entire family benefits and is far from selfish. It may even mean that breastfeeding can continue for longer. It is not uncommon to meet a parent who felt able to continue breastfeeding once night-times became easier and they felt more rested. It may be that they have more patience and energy for daytime feeding requests. It may be that night weaning triggered a return to fertility so they felt able to continue breastfeeding while trying to conceive again. It can give parents the space to be the parents they want to be.

Too often when parents ask professionals for support on night weaning, they are presented with extinction methods such as controlled crying or 'cry it out' or even a version of a gradual retreat that is very structured and prescribed. As Dr Gordon describes, parents should be supported to listen to their gut instincts about what feels right and what doesn't: 'Your instincts are better than any sleep-modification program ever written' (Gordon 2020). For parents who have practised natural-term feeding (or certainly closer to the natural term), the idea of using sleep training methods often feels profoundly uncomfortable but they may be offered little else. Underlying the offer is sometimes an implication that they have been indulgent by feeding this long and they don't just need to correct a sleep habit but 'correct' the child's belief that they will always meet their needs. Truthfully, it is possible to night wean and continue to breastfeed for many more months or years. It is possible to night wean and continue to be a responsive and gentle parent.

For parents

Lyndsey Hookway has some suggestions for parents when they are looking for a professional to support them with sleep.

> Q. If a parent wants to find a professional to support them with their child's sleep, what should they be considering?
> There are some questions that I've developed that can guide conversations when families are looking for a sleep supporter:
>
> 1) Ask about their training experience and skills supporting parents with biologically normal responsive sleep. Not all sleep supporters are created equal. What courses have they done? Do they have additional qualifications? Do you connect with them?
>
> 2) Would they try to get your baby sleeping at whatever cost or do

they sound realistic? Are they saying that normal issues can't and shouldn't be fixed?

3) Will they be promoting schedules, fixed awake windows, sleep timings? Are they talking about sleeping through the night? Are they offering a feeding routine when they have no infant feeding qualification? Are they offering a guarantee of success? Does it sound too good to be true?

4) Will they ask you to stop doing something that is meaningful to you like bedsharing, feeding to sleep, contact napping or breastfeeding?

5) What do they understand by responsiveness? Does that gel well with your understanding of the term? How will their support help you maintain responsiveness?

6) Will they ask you to leave your child or baby to cry or be in any distress on their own? Ask a specific question here. Sometimes people consider controlled crying to be gentle because it's not 'cry it out'. Ask them outright if they require you to leave your child without emotional support.

7) What will happen if you disagree with them? Do they use a range of tools or is it a one size fits all? If it's the latter, chances are if you don't like it, they will not offer an alternative or a refund. Are you allowed to try something and change your mind? Will they continue to support you? What if something isn't working? If you are worried, is it clear how you can complain?

Bottom line, if you feel like you could go out for a coffee with this person and put the world to rights, they're probably sound. If they make your stomach sink, walk away.

Chapter 6

Returning to Work

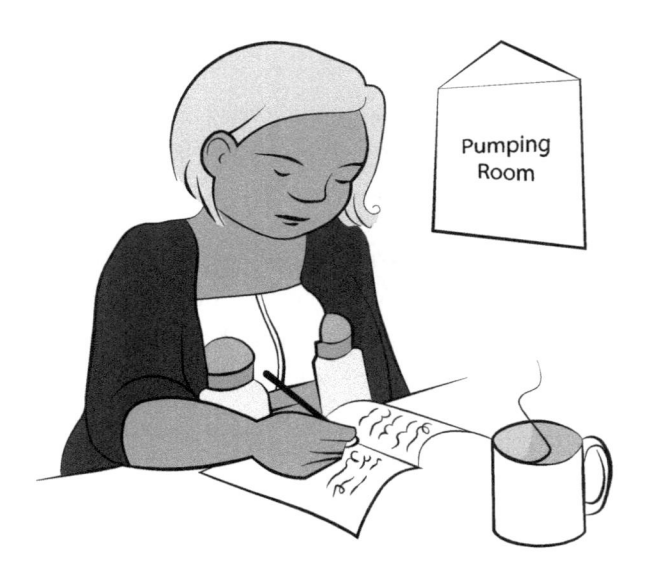

In some countries, where extended maternity/parental leave is not the norm, a discussion around returning to work while breastfeeding will have taken place in the very early days. It may even have shaped some of the very first parenting decisions made such as which breast pump was purchased in pregnancy, the gifting of a bra that allows for hands-free pumping and an expectation that a baby will need to be able to take a bottle from the very early days. If you are a professional supporting families in the USA, for example, the idea of talking to someone breastfeeding at six months about their return to work may seem faintly ludicrous, let alone ten or 12 months. Whereas in Europe, talking to someone with a six-month-old baby, or even a toddler, about breastfeeding alongside a return to work may be a more regular experience, and therefore it has a natural home in this book.

The average maternity leave in the USA is around ten weeks as the Family and Medical Leave Act (FMLA) enables around 60% of employees to take up to 12 weeks' unpaid leave (which often results as two weeks taken at the end of pregnancy and ten weeks after baby has arrived) (Bryant 2020). Some states have passed their own family leave laws but the USA remains the only OECD country without a national statutory paid parental leave. As of April 2021, this may change as President Joe Biden is proposing to introduce 12 weeks of paid leave in his American Families Plan. It's hard to fathom just how much experience differs among parents in different countries. In Estonia, mothers can continue to be paid full wages for the first 18 months of baby's life with some reduced monthly payments continuing even after that. In the UK, a full year is an option but only the first six weeks is at 90% of their usual salary, with several weeks at a reduction and nothing for the final 13 weeks. UK birthing parents are required to take a minimum of two weeks off after birth (and possibly four weeks depending on the nature of their job). Other countries also enforce compulsory leave: Mexico and Austria both enforce several weeks' leave before and after birth.

There is not only enormous variation internationally but obviously in the same city or neighbourhood too. You may support families where maternity leave and parental leave is not a realistic option for financial reasons and you will be answering questions about breastfeeding alongside paid work before colostrum has even had a chance to transition to mature milk or postnatal bleeding has stopped. One of our earliest messages will be that an early return to work is not a barrier to continued breastfeeding. In the USA, where there is not statutory maternity leave, breastfeeding rates are consistently higher than the UK where a year's leave is an option and several months of leave is common.

In the USA, according to the Centers for Disease Control and

Prevention (CDC) breastfeeding report card, exclusive breastfeeding at three months is 46.9% on a national level compared to 17% in the UK (Renfrew et al. 2011). In the USA, any breastfeeding at six months is 58.3% with breastfeeding at 12 months being 35.3%, according to the CDC report card. In the UK, at six months, 34% of babies receive some breastmilk. However, it is perhaps telling that these UK figures come from 2010 as the government's capturing of breastfeeding data in its national survey ended then. There are no UK figures at 12 months. Maybe a political will to measure and assess breastfeeding rates is connected to deeper cultural issues, but this may not be a place for that discussion. Scotland has jurisdiction over its own health matters and has historically a greater commitment to supporting breastfeeding than the UK national government (which governs English health). The Information Services Division in Scotland reports that at the 13- to 15-month review, 18% of babies are still receiving some breastmilk (Information Services Division 2019).

So while it is tempting to make a connection between extended maternity leave and breastfeeding beyond the first six months, and logic suggests that in many countries those staying at home longer are likely to breastfeed for longer, the idea that returning to work means an end to breastfeeding is not a correct assumption. It is a simple message that we can convey to parents. Not only is breastfeeding possible alongside working outside the home but it is desirable. Putting aside all the reasons why continued breastfeeding is beneficial to child and parental health, it reduces the chance that a child will be ill, and the parent will be required to be absent from work as a result. In a 1995 study of parents returning from maternity leave after an uncomplicated birth:

> Approximately 28% of the infants in the study had no illnesses; 86% of these were breast-fed and 14% were formula-fed. When illnesses occurred, 25% of all one-day maternal absences were among breast-fed babies and 75% were among the formula-fed group. (Cohen, Mrtek and Mrtek 1995)

Employers who get behind supporting breastfeeding in the workplace aren't doing so entirely out of a natural sense of generosity and affection for their employees. A breastfeed has an emotional value that goes beyond the constituents of breastmilk, antibodies and millilitres. When the parent picks their baby up at their caregiver, and they have the feed that is a special 'hello and welcome back', they are creating memories and carving out a moment of peace. They are also helping to ensure that whatever microbes their baby collected during the day, their milk will go into action creating the soldiers to keep them at bay. There also continues to be a financial incentive if the alternative is the purchase of formula milk.

As a breastfeeding supporter or health professional, you are helping a parent to visualize the rhythm of a new life. They are capable of the internet search that outlines the basics, but they want to say out loud how their personalized version of that is going to go. Sometimes, your service may simply be listening as they say out loud the shape of their working day or helping them to write it down. There are so many things to remember and so many things to think about, any conversation they have with you ideally ends in notes they can take away and refer to later.

Common questions from parents

How much milk will a baby need when they are separated?

We usually assume a rough estimate of 30 ml (1 US fl oz) for each hour of separation if a baby is around six months old (Kent *et al.* 1999; Neville *et al.* 1988). However, the minute solid food enters the equation and a baby is capable of drinking water from a cup, that may start to adjust (Dewey, Finley and Lönnerdal 1984). If a caregiver is practising responsive bottle-feeding, also known as paced bottle-feeding, they should start to get a sense of a baby's daily intake over time. There is a lot of individual variation. At six months, some babies will have an intake of 600 ml (20 US fl oz) and others will have an intake of 900 ml (30 US fl oz), so inevitably daily intake will vary. Some will be feeding throughout the night, and daytime is more about play and chatter than getting in the calories. Other babies sleep throughout the night and have a daytime mission to load up. Some ten-month-old babies will have 50% of their calorie intake from solid food and be cup experts. Others will depend on breastmilk with solid food being an occasional and unenthusiastic mouthful. An early message for parents is that it's OK to wait and see before feeling as though you must have all the answers now. You may not entirely know how pumping at work is going to go or how your breasts might feel. You may not entirely be able to predict what your baby will take when you are separated. Any plan you make now is not forever. In just a matter of weeks, their solids intake may change dramatically. When a parent is nervous, a sense of planning helps to bring a sense of control, but it may be an artificial sense if adaptation will be quickly needed. We can help give confidence by talking through options.

Does a baby have to be able to take a bottle for a parent to return to work?

This can bring a huge amount of anxiety. It can impact on the first few weeks of breastfeeding if it's felt taking a bottle is an essential. There are myths about magical windows that are when a baby MUST take a bottle, or all is lost. There are myths about the type of bottle that MUST be used alongside breastfeeding. With infant feeding, there are few 'MUSTS'. Truthfully, a baby may never take a bottle enthusiastically from the parent who breastfeeds them but acquiesce with no issue when being fed by someone else. It is also perfectly possible for a baby to never drink milk from a bottle and their parent can return to work with ease. Even from the first few weeks, that can be an option. In the early days, cup-feeding and syringe-feeding can be options. Babies may respond well to finger-feeding (using a tube feeding system taped to a finger). With both syringe-feeding and finger-feeding, baby will be semi-reclined and have a finger in contact with their palate; as they suck on a finger, they will be rewarded either by milk being drawn down through the tube or a caregiver slowly trickling milk into the corner of their mouth with a syringe.

From around four months, cup-feeding may move from the smaller infant feeding cups and on to commercial cups designed for independent drinking. In the UK, the NHS recommends moving from breast to cup and talks about 'discouraging' bottles from 12 months (NHS 2018a). This is valuable information for someone returning to work at nine or ten months who imagines bottle-feeding is a necessary requirement. For older nurslings, where only three or four feeds in 24 hours may meet their necessary intake, it may be possible for the parent to feed in the morning and at drop-off, at pick-up and in the evening, so have a baby that doesn't feed at night and needs no additional milk in the day, whether from a bottle or anything else. It is not unusual for a 12-month-old, or even a nine- or ten-month-old who enjoys solids, to not take additional milk during a working day.

How can expressed milk be stored during a working day?

A parent may have access to a fridge at work but this is by no means a requirement, and the idea of sharing a fridge with other colleagues may cause anxiety. Freshly expressed milk can be stored in an insulated cool bag with freezer blocks for up to 24 hours (Hamosh *et al.* 1996). And if room temperature is around 21°C (70°F), then six hours' storage without any kind of cooling can be fine (Eglash *et al.* 2017). If a parent is pumping more than once during a working day, this logic also suggests that re-washing and re-sterilizing pumping equipment isn't likely to be necessary, especially as we are talking about older, less vulnerable babies. If equipment has just come into contact with breastmilk, it could be stored in a Tupperware box or re-closable bag and kept cool and then re-used later and washed thoroughly in hot soapy water once the parent is home.

How much will a parent need to express during a working day?

If you provide a standard answer to this question, it's time to re-think. There is no 'everyone MUST express' every three hours or 'at least twice'. This is going to be a very individual decision. It's likely to depend on their working day: someone in a quiet office working alone may prioritize differently from a police officer or school teacher. It's likely to depend on how often a baby usually feeds in the day. If a toddler feeds once before a lunchtime nap, the pumping schedule will be different than if they graze on and off throughout the day. A parent with a smaller storage capacity who gets engorged more quickly may need to express more frequently in order to remain comfortable, reduce the risk of leaking and protect their milk supply. A parent with a larger storage capacity may not become engorged in the length of a working day and may not feel the need to express at all, especially if they have an older child who feeds less frequently. If a parent doesn't become engorged, and this means less accumulation of the FIL (feedback inhibitor of lactation) protein believed to contribute to a reduction in milk supply and less distension of the prolactin receptors (another contributing factor), supply may not be at risk at all.

A parent who has a significant freezer stash may have little need to express large quantities in the day. Although, it may be useful to have a conversation about why devoting energy to building a freezer stash in the early weeks may not always be a positive (as it may send unhelpful signals resulting in over-supply or miss an opportunity for more direct feeding or fresh milk).

Some parents may have nurslings that reverse cycle, that is, reverse typical day and night-time patterns. When babies are small, this can be distressing, but on the return to work and with older nurslings this can be useful. If a parent doesn't enjoy pumping and finds co-sleeping and night-time feeding straightforward, they may encourage their nursling to directly feed at the breast overnight and very little milk is needed during a working day, and sometimes none.

Not all parents can visualize how patterns will change as their baby gets older. At six months, when breastfeeding is their baby's entire nutrition, their pumping plans are vital. But as young as nine or ten months, a baby may breastfeed on wake-up, again when a parent sees them at the end of a working day and once at bedtime (baby's or parent's bedtime). A parent may not need to express at all at work. They may not need to store any milk. Baby may eat some solids and drink a little water when they are separated.

Not all parents appreciate that the pattern during a working week may need to be adapted. If a parent returns to direct breastfeeding at the weekend, it may be on Monday they need to express a little more for comfort after some additional supply stimulation. That need may reduce throughout the week until by Thursday or Friday, no pumping is needed at all.

How can a parent talk to an employer about their rights at work?

Each country and even local district will have their own laws and guidelines on rights at work. In the UK, ACAS (Advisory, Conciliation and Arbitration Service) provides a useful resource which outlines the rights of the breastfeeding parent in the workplace (or rather the disappointing lack of them): 'Accommodating breastfeeding employees in the workplace' (ACAS 2014).

The charity Maternity Action can provide some useful information, whether through their advice line or online factsheets, for example 'Continuing to breastfeed when you return to work' (Maternity Action 2016). Whatever the legal situation, few employers fail to appreciate that protecting an employee makes good business sense. An employee that breastfeeds beyond the first year will have very little to worry about in terms of their impact on the working day, assuming they are not working with hazardous materials. Not all employers appreciate that accommodating someone breastfeeding at 12 months is a very different story from accommodating someone breastfeeding at three months. An employer may not understand the practicalities of supporting breastfeeding or why it is in their interests to do so, and sometimes a conversation with a breastfeeding supporter, or the opportunity to ask questions (with the parent's permission), can provide reassurance. Early conversations are likely to be better than later ones. Is there a policy? Can the parent find a mentor within the workplace who has returned to work while breastfeeding?

One area that can cause some challenges is a discussion around night shifts or staying away from home when a nursling is still night feeding, especially if the breast is an important part of their falling-to-sleep routine. There may not be an easy answer to this, other than to say older nurslings are surprisingly adaptable at sometimes falling asleep in a different way when breasts are not available. And employers, and other colleagues, are surprisingly adaptable if someone feels they are unable to be away from home at their child's bedtime for what is a relatively short period of time in a career (even if you are breastfeeding an older child). Sometimes creative thinking is needed. It might be that a nursling and another carer can also attend a work trip or an employee can take a longer break to return home for bedtime and then come back to the workplace.

There is some legal precedent for an employer's responsibility to protect the breastfeeding relationship in the UK beyond the initial few months. In a 2016 case involving two easyJet cabin crew members, the court found it was indirect sex discrimination and a breach of the health and safety regulations when easyJet declined to be flexible with rosters while the women were breastfeeding. Their family doctors had written letters to state that working for longer than eight hours increased the risks of breast health problems such as engorgement and mastitis. EasyJet had offered ground work for six months but the tribunal said that employers need to continue to protect their health and safety and provide suitable alternative work for as long as they breastfeed (*Mcfarlane and Ambacher v easyJet Airline Company Limited* 2016).

In another UK case, a mother was advised by her family doctor to breastfeed for at least a year because there was a strong history of eczema in her family. She returned to work when her baby was six months old and asked to work part-time until her baby was a year old so she could continue breastfeeding around her working hours. The employer said no, but she won her case for indirect sex discrimination at an employment tribunal (Maternity Action 2016, p.5).

What else can a parent do to prepare for a return to work?

It sounds simplistic but – relax. If a parent's maternity/parental leave is limited, it should not be dominated by mental and practical preparations for returning to work. What can be useful is talking to other people who have been through it before and even finding people going through it right now. They may also be a future mentor for the parents who come after them.

> I returned to work the week my daughter turned one. I had never spent a night away from her during that time and had massively under-estimated how much she still fed, day and night. I also hadn't really used a proper pump before as my daughter would never accept a bottle. I worked as a university lecturer in a different city, and had to stay overnight (fortunately with my mum) at least once a week. The first overnight trip was a disaster! By late afternoon on the first day my boobs were rock solid and I was in agony, and all I had brought with me was my little silicone Haakaa pump. Honestly, I don't know what I was thinking, I had put off thinking about going back to work until the last possible moment and just hadn't really thought through what it would mean for us as a family nor for me as an individual. I tried to use it in the toilets at work in the middle of the day, which was hilarious but ineffective, and ended up having to leave a work meeting because I was so uncomfortable. I then spent an evening

hand expressing in the bath before enduring the next day. I literally ran off the train and stuffed my boob into her mouth when I got home. I remembered to bring my pump the following week but the only place I could use to pump was my office and I was pretty embarrassed by the noise. Support from my workplace was basically non-existent, and the only facility for storing milk was a dirty fridge shared by staff and students, so I ended up throwing it away, though this still involved smuggling it to the loos (also shared with students) and flushing it away. Luckily this was at a point in time where I'd met my breastfeeding goals so it did not affect my confidence or ability to feed my daughter, but had I returned earlier it would have been disastrous. In terms of how my daughter and partner coped – she was upset that I wasn't there and they both had a pretty restless night (she was a terrible sleeper until recently, even after night weaning about a year after I returned to work), but they adjusted and it worked OK for the 15 months I was back at work before Covid.

~ *(Sarah Pett)*

I returned to work with both Florence and Paula when they were ten months old, and my partner stayed home for a while on parental leave. This meant he could bring our baby to my workplace for a lunchtime feed in the first few weeks and this was extremely helpful for everyone. They never got on with bottles, so he offered some expressed milk or formula in a cup, but neither of them drank much milk in my absence. They would make up for it in the evenings and nights. I tried expressing at work after having Paula and found it pretty soul-destroying. Sitting in a dark, small room on my own, during my lunch break, taking 20 minutes to get a tiny bit of milk. Storing my milk was difficult because it turned sour and my baby wouldn't take much, or anything, from a bottle, so it was a pretty pointless exercise. I only expressed for a couple of months, just to ensure I wasn't engorged. My line manager did not offer much empathy or support when I suffered with sleep deprivation with Florence. She

> was aware that I was still breastfeeding and suggested I 'manage the sleep situation' to improve my mental and physical health. This advice was not very helpful to me, obviously, and I stopped looking for support from her and found it in other places by joining the local La Leche League group. On days off, I would breastfeed my babies as usual, on demand, and I never had any issues with supply engorgement, or mastitis.
>
> ~ *(Saskia)*

When Saskia is talking about her milk turning sour, she may be referring to a phenomenon where some parents have high levels of lipase enzyme which can make storing milk very challenging. Milk can be scalded before freezing.

> I was lucky to be able to take a relatively long maternity leave and returned to work when Keir was almost 14 months old. I had been very anxious about how he would get on at nursery without breastfeeding during the day, particularly with naps. He had always been breastfed to sleep/wake at nap times and often only slept on or beside me. I shouldn't have worried so much – he generally napped very well at nursery (I still have no idea how!). As he was over 12 months, he drank water or cows' milk from a cup during the day. As soon as we were reunited after a long day of work/nursery, we had a big breastfeed and cuddle. It felt like a relief to be together again and it was a huge comfort to both of us. We co-slept and I did find that he increased feeding during the night at this time. For the first few months, I would express a couple of times a day at work (using a manual pump or by hand) for my own comfort. I didn't have any need to save and store this milk. My body seemed to adjust really well and after a while I didn't need to express any more. I am about to return to work part-time for the second time, and this time I feel

more confident that we'll be able to navigate the change and I'll be able to continue feeding both my boys.

~ *(Hannah)*

I returned to work once my daughter was one year old. It was very hard mentally, which I wasn't prepared for nor expected. I was worried about how the childcare setting would get my daughter to sleep that wasn't on the breast. I realized how quickly children adapt to new ways of sleeping with different people. It also had a significant impact on my sleep. The change to not having milk constantly 'on open tap' meant that our nights became more interrupted and my daughter used to drink then to make up for what she didn't get throughout the wake hours, both in terms of comfort and closeness with Mummy but also in terms of nutrients, I guess. I had to nip out of the bedroom so early in the mornings and often leave before my daughter was up, which was really hard and I felt a lot of 'Mummy guilt' for that. Whenever I could, we had long morning cuddles and feeds and also long evening ones and she was very upset when I wasn't available and 'only' Daddy was there to comfort. At work, I decided not to pump as it was too complicated to have the milk cooled for the entire journey time from work which was long, let alone all the set-up at work and storage there. My daughter was very happy with cows' milk when at nursery, and when I picked her up, my breasts were plump full so it was always a relief to feed her as soon as we got through the door.

~ *(Eve)*

Nat is a health professional who works some night shifts:

In hindsight, I worried far too much in advance as I was going back on shifts when she was one year old and was terrified she wouldn't cope without boobs at night (as she fed to sleep and fed through the night). My work acknowledged I was coming back as a breastfeeding mum but I think I was an unusual case as most people stopped before returning. I went to a workshop for returning to work which made me feel more anxious and I contacted a friend who worked shifts and breastfed and she was really helpful. If I could go back and speak to myself back then I would not have tried to plan and research as much, as it all turned out fine (and just like everyone said, my partner and baby found their own way and we're FINE).

~ *(Nat)*

For parents

The first few weeks are often a blur for new parents. The learning curve is steep, and you survive day to day – remembering to shower and put food in the fridge for yourself if you are lucky. For those parents still in the middle of that blur, the thought of the eventual return to work can be one that provokes anxiety. You can't imagine how it will feel to leave this new special person in your life. How do you cope with drop-offs to childcare and getting back to work after potentially several night-wakings? What do you do if you don't want to give up breastfeeding?

What are some strategies that will help with a return to work?

1) *Don't think about it.*

    That doesn't mean literally never let it enter your mind but there is a balance. My message is just that if you are going to take six months, eight months or a year off work and you spend several months of that stressing about the return to work, you will be seriously missing out. STOP yourself thinking about it too much. If you stare at your gorgeous three-month-old and think fleetingly, 'How can I ever leave you?' (which is how nature very much wants you to feel), that is fair enough. But if you spend chunks of your parental leave feeling anxious and worrying about practicalities, you will be wasting the special time you do have together.

This time is precious. Your baby now is not going to be the same person when you return to work. They will sleep differently, feed differently, and interact differently. You will not be leaving THIS baby but an older one. Get your childcare sorted (which you may well have thought about in pregnancy anyway), and other than that, there's not too much more to do. If you intend to express milk at work, it's a good idea to write to your employer about two months before you go back to work to talk about arrangements. And then just carry on as normal. If your four-month-old baby won't take a bottle and that starts you panicking because you must go back to work at eight months, don't think about it. An eight-month-old baby can breastfeed when you are with them in the morning and evening, take a sippy cup, drink from an open cup – you will have options. And a four-month-old baby that refuses a bottle may not if you try again after leaving it for a few weeks. It's very easy to set yourself into a panic when the truth is that things usually work out with the right information and the right support.

2) *As mentioned, speak to your employer.*
Your rights will vary according to where you live.

The recommendation is that you inform them that you will be returning to work while feeding your baby so they have a chance to assess your health and safety and what provisions you may need. In the UK, your employers are required to keep you safe. They also have a legal requirement to allow you to 'rest' if you are breastfeeding. In the UK, there is not a clearly set out legal right to express breastmilk at work and it's important you talk to your employer so they have advanced warning and you can come to an arrangement. Some employees need to have break times re-organized or a room found. Although there is no 'legal right' most employers understand that it is in their interests to try and meet your needs and provide you with facilities. Case law has also established that employers do have a requirement to keep you safe – which means not putting you at risk of breast health problems. Your morale also matters, and a baby receiving your milk is less likely to suffer from illness, meaning less time off work for you. However, employers will be more likely to be accommodating if you give them warning and explain your needs clearly. We assume that supporting breastfeeding alongside a return to work automatically means we are talking about expressing milk and pumping breaks. In many cases, direct breastfeeding in the day can also be facilitated and is more convenient, especially for those who may have difficulty using a pump or storing milk. You may prefer your child to be cared for near your workplace so you have the journey together and then you can visit in your lunch break.

3) *Talk through your schedule with a breastfeeding counsellor or lactation consultant.*

    Breastfeeding support is not just for people with problems with positioning and attachment. It's common for a parent to come along a few weeks before their return to work to talk about how they hope to organize their feeding and pumping schedule and how to organize things practically. You could also ring a breastfeeding helpline. They may help you reflect on your options or consider things you've not thought about.

4) *Practise pumping.*

    Is the breast pump you are using at home something you are familiar with? Do you have a backup if you need to pump at work? Is it worth sourcing a double pump if time is an issue or even hiring a hospital-grade electric breast pump for a few months which can just stay at work? In the UK, you'd be looking at paying around £47 a month and you can hire from companies such as Ardo Breast Pumps.

    There are tricks such as preparing the breast using massage and warm compresses. And we know that if you finish a pumping session using hand expression techniques, you can increase your output considerably.

It's also not a bad idea to build up a bit of a freezer stash before you go back. If you start pumping for one extra session each day and storing that in a freezer bag (store them flat and build up layers of thin flat bags which defrost more easily and take up less space), you will have some wiggle room if you need it. It's not entirely predictable how pumping will go at work and some find that their pumping output decreases towards the end of the week and then a weekend of normal breastfeeding boosts it back up again. If you have that freezer stash, it will take away some of the anxiety. However, if your nursling is older and eating solids and drinking water, you may have little reason for storing milk at all.

5) *Get your kit.*

So, you need a pump and some bottles, and some breastmilk storage bags. What else? Surprisingly not much. You don't need to store freshly expressed breastmilk in the fridge at work if you don't want to. You can have a freezer block and an insulated bag and put any expressed milk in there. It is fine in that for 24 hours. If you store it like that at work, put it in the fridge when you get home, then that milk can be given to your baby's carer for the next day.

It's also important to note there is a lack of evidence to suggest you need to wash and sterilize the pump between all pumping sessions. Breastmilk is fine at room temperature for up to six hours. So, do you need to wash a pump between your 11 am pumping session and your 2 pm one? Some working parents use a technique called 'wet-bagging', putting a pump in a plastic bag between sessions and then putting it back in the fridge. Then simply take it out next time and wipe any wet parts with paper kitchen towel if you don't fancy cold drips against you! This also saves precious time. More research is needed on the finer details of milk storage and washing pumps, so we need to apply what we know from the studies we do have.

6) *Feed your baby directly when you can.*

Your supply is more likely to be maintained if you breastfeed when you get the chance. Is your childcare near work or home? Could you visit your baby at lunchtime? Could you work from home for one day a week for the first few weeks? You could breastfeed early in the morning, then once more at drop-off, once more at pick-up and again at home later in the evening. Those four feeds could be enough breastmilk overall for a baby of eight months or more. You may not need to be carrying bottles back and forth. And breastfeeding at the weekends and during holidays will help to boost your supply.

Here are the stories of two mothers:

Phoebe

Phoebe is returning to work at ten months. She is a graphic designer and works from home with some client visits necessary around London. Her daughter breastfeeds around four times in 24 hours and enjoys solids which she started at six months. Phoebe doesn't enjoy pumping and finds it difficult so would rather avoid it if possible. She finds a childminder who lives near her home. Phoebe breastfeeds at 8.30 am and drops her daughter at the childminder. If she is working from home, she visits at lunchtime for another breastfeed. She then collects her daughter at around 4 pm and takes her home to breastfeed at 6 pm and around 11 pm. While her daughter is at the childminder, she eats solid food and drinks water. The childminder doesn't give her milk. When Phoebe has a client visit, she sometimes hand expresses for a few minutes into a plastic bag when she can grab a private moment. This is just to stay comfortable when she feels particularly engorged. This will help to reduce her risk of blocked ducts and mastitis and help to maintain her supply. She doesn't keep the milk. Phoebe continues breastfeeding her daughter until she is

18 months old. At the end she is only breastfeeding in the morning and evening and Phoebe doesn't feel the need to use any hand expression when they are separated.

Catherine

Catherine is returning to work at eight months. Her son breastfeeds around six times in 24 hours. He started solids at six months. He doesn't particularly like bottles and usually only takes around 2 oz max (60 ml) in one sitting. Catherine finds that he will take more milk from an open cup called a doidy cup. He will also be more likely to take it if she mixes the breastmilk with ripe banana and makes a smoothie. She works four days a week (and at 12 months will go back to being full time). Catherine is a teacher. Her headteacher has struggled to find her a private room for pumping but has given her the key to the medical room, and if that is in use, she uses a stock cupboard and she has told staff that when her scarf is on the door, please knock. Usually the medical room is empty. Her colleagues have agreed to relieve her of playground duty while she is breastfeeding. She breastfeeds her son at 5.45 am and again at 7.30 am at the childminder. She arrives at school at 8 am. She expresses at 10.45 am during morning break. She expresses for ten minutes. She expresses again at lunchtime for 15 minutes and at around 4 pm for another ten minutes. She prefers to use a double pump as her pumping time is restricted. She remains at school for meetings and lesson preparation and collects her son at around 6 pm. She breastfeeds him at 7 pm and 10 pm. He wakes to feed between 1 am and 2 am and Catherine is happy for that to continue for the time being as he feeds and goes back to sleep quickly.

With the childminder, her son takes around 3 oz of breastmilk in his smoothie, 2 oz mixed into a porridge and another 1–2 oz from

> his doidy cup. She also makes sure his solids contain good sources of fats and calcium. Sometimes she struggles to pump in her breaks as she really needs to continue working. She finds herself dipping into her freezer stash, and as time goes on, the childminder sometimes uses formula to make up the porridge. On the weekends and on her day off, he breastfeeds more frequently.

Working and continuing to feed your child breastmilk are not incompatible. With modern electric breast pumps and using breastfeeding support available locally, it's never been easier.

If your child is beyond 12 months, it can sometimes feel more challenging to assert your rights and have conversations with your employer where you prioritize the needs of your family. If you are asked to travel for your work and you have to explain that your two-year-old co-sleeps and feeds through the night, and you would rather not make that trip, that can feel exposing. Society is more accepting that accommodations are necessary when we are talking about younger babies. Society isn't always so patient as the years go by. As a parent feeding an older child, you are used to being brave and these are the conversations where we may need to be the bravest. You are not just advocating for yourself but for your child who doesn't have access to this conversation. You are also advocating for the generations of parents who will come after you. It is always worth asking. There is no harm in making a request. You can make reference to your own physical health: those feeding older children don't always find expressing easier. You can offer another time. You can explain it would bring some challenges for your family. There is some legal precedent in the UK for employers having to make accommodations for older nurslings as mentioned earlier in the chapter. Having said all that, if things don't go as you wish, and you don't have time to wait for the results of an industrial tribunal, it is surprising how adaptable older nurslings can be. There are working parents who breastfeed for years alongside regular travel, night shifts and long hours. The night-time nursling who co-sleeps and is attached to you on and off the entire night is more capable than we might always appreciate. They can adapt their sleeping strategies to the circumstances and understand that different adults can provide different things.

> I returned to work when J was just over a year. I feel like continuing to breastfeed once back at work was really helpful for both of us. It gave her the comfort and nutrition she needed after a busy day at nursery/with grandparents, as well as being the easiest way of getting her off to sleep. And it gave me a much-needed way of re-connecting with her after being apart all day. I had deliberately started reducing breastfeeds from around nine months old (which in retrospect I don't think I would do again), so by the time I was back at work my supply had dropped enough that I never felt particularly engorged or the need to pump at work. However, I was always glad to get home and feed her! Breastfeeding whilst working was very straightforward for us and not something I ever particularly thought much about.
>
> ~ *(Naomi Dow)*

Chapter 7

Nursing Manners and Communicating Limits

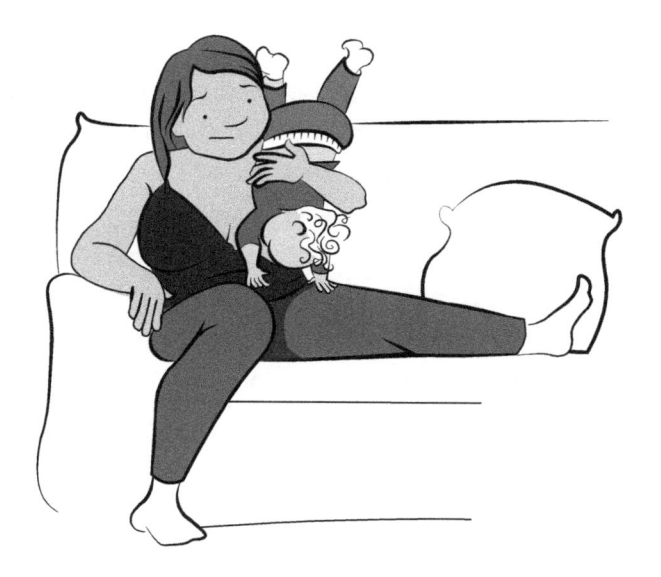

The subject of nursing manners is a topic most professionals will not even have considered an area for major concern. What are we even talking about? Does it mean asking nicely and saying 'thank you' afterwards? In fact, it's about encouraging an older nursling to feed in a way that's comfortable for their parent and respectful of them as a separate person. This may include not stretching the nipple, not contorting into positions that may be frustrating and not fiddling with other parts of the parent's body. Even if an explanation is given, it can be hard to see what the problem is if you haven't spent a lot of time with an older nursling. Why don't parents just stop it from happening? Why would someone tolerate something that is uncomfortable or painful? Just tell them 'no' or stop the feed! Unfortunately it is not that straightforward, and struggling with nursing manners is not a symptom of weak parenting skills.

Often uncomfortable nursing manners creep very slowly towards being a problem. A little hand that begins to pull at your skin might even be endearing in the very early days. It's a sign that the pincer grip is emerging. The smile that accompanies it may even be worth it. It won't be for every feed, just now and again. Who wants to be disciplining a baby of three or four months who barely understands that it is their hand in front of their nose? When a baby is approximately four months old, it's common for them to enter a phase where they are very distractible in the day. This phase may last several months. They may reverse cycle and want to take more calories overnight and feeds during the day may be reluctantly acquiesced to when they are particularly hungry or thirsty. When a parent finally does get a baby to attach and swallow, the idea of taking them off to discuss what they are doing with their fingernails does not feel instinctive. So when a parent does finally become conscious of the fact that their child's behaviour at the breast is a problem, it may have been a lifetime in the making and confusing for a child to understand what the problem even is. When a child pulls at your shirt to ask for a breastfeed, it's often useful. A baby doing it is delightful, but when it becomes an older nursling, perhaps in public one day for the first time accompanied with frustration, it can suddenly feel less welcome.

> Nursing manners was the biggest challenge we faced. It was more or less an ongoing battle to get Fin to feed in a respectful way and stop the nursing gymnastics and tugging at clothing. That was the hardest thing for me as I started to feel a bit out of control of the

breastfeeding relationship, and if things weren't working for me then it was hard to communicate that with my two-year-old.

~ *(Rachel, who fed Finlay for two and a half years)*

I had a zero tolerance approach to biting, pinching, twiddling, switch nursing, fiddling, etc. from a very early age. They make my skin crawl and I found them all totally unacceptable. I don't remember exactly when I instigated nursing manners but I suspect it was under six months. I told J a firm 'no, thank you, Mummy doesn't like that', and if she continued then I ended the feed. She didn't starve before she learned!

~ *(Naomi)*

Both my kids 'fumble' a LOT which can get very annoying at times. I used teething necklaces a little, and as the language skills increased, explaining helped. My daughter used to twist the nipple of my other breast all the time and would get upset when I wouldn't let her. My son digs his fingernails into my neck and pinches and scratches a lot. This too will pass is my motto.

~ *(Eve)*

If you spend ten minutes in a social media group where breastfeeding older children is the norm, you'll come across the topic of toddler nipple twiddling which is one specific concern in the nursing manners arena.

Toddlers enjoy fiddling generally: the little plastic figure in their hand, the toy car, car keys, glasses. It's how they explore their world, develop their fine motor skills, calm themselves and occupy themselves. And when they are breastfeeding, the other nipple often looks like another appealing button. Some stroke, some twist, some pull, some rub between a finger and thumb, some twiddle to get to sleep. If a toddler enjoyed poking their parent in the eye during breastfeeding, it's unlikely they would tolerate it many times. Imagine if a child's favourite thing was fiddling with someone else's eyelashes? Imagine the sticky little fingers and teeny fingernails. Parents wouldn't hesitate to say things like: 'I don't like that. That hurts my eye. That makes me feel uncomfortable. Please don't touch my eye.'

We need to encourage parents to feel empowered to express their feelings when nipple twiddling similarly bothers them. I think because it's the nipple, parents somehow feel as though it's part of breastfeeding. You might read something about how the nursling is stimulating a let-down reflex and a parent could think, 'It's natural so I'm stuck.' Nipple twiddling, and other nursing habits such as skin stroking or tummy button excavating, can be comforting for a toddler and help them to calm and settle into a feed. To resist that can lead to protest, a disrupted feed and a nap not happening – reducing oxytocin at a moment when you want to get some oxytocin happening in your child. As it gives the child calm and comfort, parents often feel they have to tolerate it, in a world where parents are all too used to putting their own needs in second place.

When we talk to parents about nursing manners, we can support them to understand that their body autonomy matters too. I say this a lot when I talk about breastfeeding older children: this is their first intimate relationship. This is a model for how important relationships are going to go in their life and it's about far more than milk delivery and about far more than their comfort. Parents are teaching their nurslings slowly and gradually that they are a person too. Child-led weaning is not a scenario where empathy has been removed. Natural-term breastfeeding is not about teaching your child that your feelings don't matter. That would be a waste of vital life lessons. Most parents are talking to young children about their body autonomy. More than ever before, we are encouraging children to use the correct terms to describe their body parts and we are no longer forcing children to kiss distant relatives. In the UK, the NSPCC (National Society for the Prevention of Cruelty to Children) has had the PANTS campaign for nearly a decade (NSPCC 2021). It's a way to talk to young children about body autonomy and protect them against future abuse. The P means Privates are Private! The A means Always Remember Your Body Belongs to You! The N is No Means No!

Nursing Manners and Communicating Limits

The T is Talk About Secrets that Upset You! The S is Speak Up, Someone Can Help! When we are establishing boundaries around nursing manners and breastfeeding, parents are modelling the same principles they wish for their children. Not to say that if they have allowed nipple twiddling to linger, their children are at risk of abuse, but that parents should feel empowered to prioritize themselves in conversations which do have a wider impact on their child's feelings about consent and respect.

It may sound trite – but not every breastfeed is life-changing. Not every breastfeed is motivated by profound, magnificent, respect-at-all-costs urges. One parent described how during the Covid-19 lockdown, she noticed her nursling asked more simply out of boredom. She had become 'the biscuit tin'. Her son was bored and looking for something to do, just as adults might grab a snack when they weren't really that hungry. Should we ensure we never refuse feeds like those? What about the feeds that come just because we're on a work call and they want some attention? Or we're occupied with something else and they want our focus? Some of these needs can be met in different ways and it isn't a betrayal of breastfeeding to say so.

Setting limits is not just about dealing with nursing manners, it is about the heart of negotiating a breastfeeding relationship. There is a spectrum of options between allowing a child to breastfeed whenever they wish to and full weaning. Not all parents are affected by more playful feeds in the same way.

> We definitely have gymnastic feeds. Lu will get into a brilliant position and stay there for the entire session. If he's really tired he's very relaxed whilst feeding, but if it's mid playtime then he loves to twiddle my hair, pop a finger in my mouth, pop a finger up my nostrils, generally have a laugh. So our nursing manners aren't too great then, but I don't mind. It's our time to relax and have a giggle.
>
> ~ (Michelle)

During the Covid-19 pandemic, many parents breastfeeding toddlers and older children struggled with nurslings at home who were constantly asking for access to the breast. We need to give the message that nursing manners extends beyond pinching hands. It means having kindness when the breasts are in the middle of an important meeting or the breasts are tired, or the breasts need to go and get a drink of water for themselves. Even from a young age, it's OK to talk about the need to wait. Even when time is only beginning to be understood. It's OK to say, 'Do you mind if we just snuggle for a bit or read a book as my breasts/milkies/milk-milk need a bit of a rest?' Parents are teaching a vital lesson about being open with feelings and how those in loving relationships can express vulnerabilities and the need for give-and-take and compromise.

None of this is incompatible with being a breastfeeding advocate and a passionate supporter of natural-term breastfeeding. If we think child-led weaning means parents are never ever allowed to refuse, we may be dissuading others from continuing to breastfeed in the longer term. Every time we tell a parent that child-led breastfeeding means no restrictions from the parent at all and the parent must respond to every request for breastfeeding with no limits, we are potentially shutting down older babies breastfeeding for longer and perpetuating the myth that breastfeeding means you can't be a normal person with frustrations and bad days and your own goals and desires.

What might help if a parent has a Guinness World Record Breaker older nursling? What can we suggest to parents?

1) Speak openly with the nursling. Be honest. Parents can say that they love breastfeeding, and milkies is special and helps to make babies and children strong and clever, but sometimes they need a rest. Just a short one. Milkies will be along again soon. They don't have to stretch the truth and create some biological excuse. They don't have to pretend they need time to make more milk. It's just OK to say how they feel. I have met parents of three- and four-year-olds who are

struggling and will do everything (including putting band-aids on nipples) rather than just try and share how they feel. We can admit to being tired. We can admit to needing to concentrate on something else. It may be helpful to say 'We can't have milk now' rather than 'You can't have milk now.' This implies that the delay means they are both missing out and in this together rather than one person refusing the request of another.

2) Some of this is about the nursling looking to control their world but the world feels out of control. Their speech is developing and their understanding of communication. They ask for a breastfeed and it happens and that's magic. What else may fulfil that desire? Can they 'ask for a book'? It's sometimes said that reading a book together is more like breastfeeding for a toddler than most other activities. If they can't read at that moment, make a book waiting room. They can pile up the books they want you to read next, in the order they want them. Or what about a toy waiting room? Or some cards with pictures on that show favourite activities and a board where they can stick up the next request?

3) They may be thirsty. Do they have a cup station they can reach and use independently?

4) If a parent is working on a task at home, and trying to care for their nursling at the same time, what short activities give them 15-minute bursts of being able to work? In an office, we regularly take short breaks to grab tea, talk to a colleague, even just pick up our phones and scroll. It's OK for focused work at home to only be in relatively short bursts. Use a timer to show them time passing. The app 'Forest – stay focused' allows a parent to plant a cyber-tree that then gradually grows over the time they have set in advance. The nursling can come back and check on the device to see how the tree is growing. Is the tree fully grown so now it's time for a breastfeed? Or a chance to read a book?

5) A parent can grant a breastfeed but on their own terms. It can be 'count to ten' (counting slowly or quickly depending on how they are feeling). Or an older child can 'buy' a breastfeed by trading a bracelet or a toy. 'Here are five plastic spoons/coins/dinosaurs. We're going to play milkies shop. When you want a breastfeed, you can buy one. But you've only got five until lunchtime/dinnertime/I finish this piece of work.' It's amazing how long they will hang on to the last one. They feel in control knowing it's in reserve. It's still their choice when to 'spend' it.

No one has to be the 'perfect' parent who constantly puts themselves second. Finding compromises, strategies and sometimes saying 'Not right now' is healthy for both members of the dyad. If we have explicit conversations with parents about setting limits and managing expectations and if families can talk openly with us about the challenges of breastfeeding older children, it's likely many more will be able to reach their goals.

Those breastfeeding older children commonly say they don't feel they are 'allowed' to complain. If they do talk about struggles, they are often met with 'Well, you chose to breastfeed this long' or 'Perhaps you should stop now' or 'Maybe this is your body telling you that you are ready to stop. Do you know that tiger mothers in the wild…'

Often the parent didn't want a story about tiger mothers pushing their nurslings away being 'natural', they wanted empathy and possibly some practical suggestions. If the only suggestion is 'stop breastfeeding', that's a problem.

> Nursing manners has been a challenge. My daughter is very strong willed and rough, and has spent a lot of time pulling at my clothes and kicking/hitting/biting me when I refuse. She is an inveterate nipple twiddler and can get angry when asked to stop/offered an alternative like a toy. She also has very advanced language for her age, and has

started to try and persuade me into giving her booby. I have found most advice says just to be firm and persevere and they'll lose interest in x after a while, but this has not proved to be the case with her. The only exception is in the middle of the night – it took a long time but she now comes into our bed and has a cuddle and falls straight asleep rather than ask for boob.

~ *(Sarah Pett)*

Florence is now five, so we've gone from nursing on demand to an arrangement that works for us both, which changed from nursing around the clock to two times a day (when she was three), to once a day (from around when she was four). She will often ask to nurse more often, mostly because she sees her little sister Paula nurse more often, but I don't let her. When nursing an older child it's important to think about your own needs. They're no longer newborns and if you're uncomfortable you can and should do something about it. So I will ask them to change position or to stop if it is painful or uncomfortable for me. I also ask them not to stop and start every two seconds to chat, because this causes an annoying sensation for me. It is getting harder and harder for them not to chat though, now they are two and five!

~ *(Saskia)*

When my eldest son was 18 months old, I conceived my second child. I knew that breastfeeding in pregnancy could be difficult but I probably wasn't prepared for how difficult it would be. Feeding in the first three months of pregnancy was very painful. I had sensitive nipples and feeding was very uncomfortable. Then, around between three and four months, I stopped producing milk. Around the same time my son got a cold though and for three days he stopped feeding. I thought that he'd stopped feeding forever and I was very, very upset. I already felt like having a second child was going to turn his life upside down and the fact that he stopped breastfeeding felt like the first example of that. I remember feeling horribly guilty about not being able to feed him, even though he seemed OK about it. But a few days later, he decided that he would feed again, and that was then the start of about three months of dry feeding which was really very, very difficult. I went to a La Leche League meeting for help and, for the first time, people talked to me about setting boundaries with breastfeeding. I think the last time I'd got any kind of support for breastfeeding my son was a lot younger and all anyone ever talked about was 'feeding on demand'. This was the first time anyone really talked to me about feeding older babies and about setting boundaries. I suddenly realized that breastfeeding had to work for me too if we were going to continue. I started reducing feeds to just a few minutes on each side. I would sing a song, and when the song was over he would stop feeding. Some days I would sing very quickly indeed! Eventually I started producing colostrum and that eased the pain a bit. I experienced aversions some days, especially as my bump got bigger and I found sitting to feed less comfortable, but I remember some good times too, as I could feel my baby kick as I nursed his big brother.

~ (Becky)

For parents

Of course, you are a person too and it's OK to sometimes need to put your needs and wishes first. This isn't even 'being selfish', this is teaching your nursling about being a human being who cares for others. When breastfeeding starts out, they don't even realize you are a separate person. And often, we don't feel like a separate person. But as the months and then the years go by, that changes and it should change. We have times when we have to do something else. We have times when we have to care for someone else. We have times when we have to care for ourselves. We have times when we don't feel like breastfeeding.

Too often we think that the phrase often used in conjunction with natural-term breastfeeding, 'Don't offer, don't refuse', means that to 'refuse' is a betrayal of breastfeeding. But refusal (or let's call it 'negotiation' instead) is a cherished opportunity to teach that humans in this world become better humans when they care about others.

An 18-month-old, or even a three-year-old, is going to struggle with genuine empathy. They are often self-centred in a positive and wonderful way. But how does that phase end? Not by some magical delivery from fairies at around five or six or eight or nine years old. It happens slowly slowly. Even newborns react to a human face in distress. Day by day, piece by piece, a little brain changes and gets that others have feelings too.

Breastfeeding is a wonderful tool for teaching the skills that are at the heart of being a human. When you say, 'I don't like it when you fiddle with my other breast', you are helping to make a person who will form healthy relationships decades from now.

There are some practical tips that might help:

- You can tuck a piece of cloth or something textured into your clothing and encourage fiddling with that as an alternative. There are some new toys designed to be used for fidgeting that may even have nipple-like buttons.

- Offer a knitted breast, or even a silicone one.

- Move their hand to a different place with a gentle and repetitive phrase and be consistent.

- Let them say one 'hello' and then give them a choice about where the fiddling will continue: do you want my bra clip or your nose? Do you want red flannel or shirt button? You can also give them a choice about whether to feed or fiddle and explain that both can't happen at the same time.

Vanisha is feeding Munch who is now four:

> Munch was a big fan of twiddling but my aversion kicked in and we have an arrangement now, they can either drink or twiddle, not both. Munch always chooses to drink, thank goodness. When overtired or unwell, Munch will become quite assertive and sometimes insistent about nursing. However, I explain that it is not always convenient if I am busy. I find open conversations and clear boundaries helps Munch understand that nursing is not always readily available and that they may need to wait a few minutes.
>
> ~ *(Vanisha)*

Dealing with twiddling and struggling with nursing manners can be particularly challenging if you are dealing with breastfeeding aversion or agitation.

Nursing aversion and agitation are challenges that may arise for the first time when breastfeeding an older child. As Zainab Yate describes in her book *When Breastfeeding Sucks: What You Need to Know About Nursing Aversion and Agitation*:

> It is more serious than feeling tetchy a few times while breastfeeding. Having aversion can mean battling against what your body and part of your mind is telling you to do ('get this kid off me') and it can create a constant emotional burden that includes guilt and shame about feeling the way you do when you feed. (Yate 2020, p.12)

You may simultaneously want to continue breastfeeding while also hating breastfeeding. Some parents experience aversion during only some days of their menstrual cycle, or during periods of pregnancy, or with every feed for extended periods without any obvious trigger. It can help to know simply that aversion exists. It is powerful to know you are not alone. Zainab Yate's website (www.breastfeedingaversion.com) and the accompanying Facebook support group may be helpful. There can be some practical changes, such as distraction, that reduce the symptoms; Yate describes parents getting relief from holding an ice cube or watching TV. Improving the latch is also crucial as a latch with an older child which is shallow, and perhaps results in teeth grazing, can be a trigger. Improving hydration, considering dietary supplements or mindfulness techniques can also be valuable.

> Breastfeeding aversion is torture. I felt like my skin was crawling, and every ounce of my body screamed for the feeding to stop. It is such an unpleasant feeling that even the thought of it makes me want to gag. Finding a solution to the aversion takes time, but for me taking time out, getting more sleep, and feeding one child at a time helped.
>
> ~ *(Millie)*

Kathryn, who is a breastfeeding mother and an IBCLC herself:

> Aversion is awful. You don't want to stop breastfeeding. But you also can't physically stand breastfeeding. It makes you feel incredibly guilty. I started experiencing feelings of aversion at around 18 months with my last child. I noticed it was worst about two weeks before my period, so I think it was triggered by ovulation. But it also began to happen in between as well. There were some feeds where I could stand my baby being on the breast for a short period. It made my skin crawl and made me want to throw him across the room. It was incredibly difficult. The night feeds and bedtime feeds were the worst. I started on a magnesium supplement which helped a little. But I decided in order to continue breastfeeding, I needed to change something. Now when I'm supporting families with this I always suggest to work out which are the most difficult feeds, and either stop or limit these first before stopping completely. It often

> means parents can continue to feed longer and oftentimes really don't want to stop completely. So first I limited the length of the night feeds, encouraging my baby to stop before fully feeding back to sleep. We had a short feed, I would count and say we were finishing and then cuddle him tight; I found if I turned him to face away from me he was less likely to want to latch back on. This worked well and I found it doable. Then at a later date, when he was over two years, this also became intolerable so I fully night weaned. He still woke but was OK with a cuddle, a big feed in the morning and a short one as part of the bedtime routine. We continued with these feeds for a long time. I truly think that limiting the feeds and then night weaning meant I could continue to breastfeed longer. He eventually stopped just before he was four with some mutual negotiation.
>
> ~ *(Kathryn)*

Far from the message of 'Don't refuse' (and isn't 'refuse' such a loaded word suggesting something about the person 'refusing' that is immoveable and unempathic?), refusal is part of successful parenting. By demonstrating that we are people with feelings and needs and demands on our time, and encouraging our little ones to hang on and learn impulse control, we are taking valuable teaching moments.

For autistic parents and other parents who have issues with sensory processing, nursing manners and dealing with twiddling can bring additional challenges. Autistic parents are likely to have a good understanding of strategies that they may find helpful and to understand when they are reaching their own limits. You should be reassured that just because you are now caring for a baby it doesn't mean that you should be expected to be able to put your feelings and reactions to one side. Sometimes we need to centre ourselves as parents and that makes us better parents.

Motherhood and parenthood feel like the lands of sacrifice. We are constantly absorbing the message that our feelings come second (or further down the line). If we have made a choice to continue with

Nursing Manners and Communicating Limits

breastfeeding, we sometimes feel as though we have signed up to some sort of deal where we have to pretend it's all wonderful. We're not supposed to want to make restrictions. We're betraying the God of natural-term breastfeeding if we do.

This is not true. If the nipple twiddling is uncomfortable for you, end it today. If it crept up on you as a problem and you tolerated it last week or even yesterday, you are allowed to change your mind. You are allowed to remove your consent as you would have the right in any other situation involving your own body. On a practical note, this means more oxytocin and more milk flow and an improved breastfeeding experience for all. It also means your mental health and the ability to see a breastfeeding session as a positive experience is elevated. It could even extend your child's opportunity for more days, weeks or months of feeding because you'll be happier to continue.

If your toddler was poking you in the eye, you'd say 'no, thanks'. They might protest. They might get cross. You'd still say 'no, thanks'. If they want to fiddle, there are infinite other options that give you agency over your other nipple. Toddler twiddling is not something you have to put up with because your feelings aren't the priority.

Natural-term breastfeeding is about more than antibodies, protein, vitamin A or even comfort. It's a world where you have a fast-track way to create a little human filled with empathy and kindness. Use that opportunity.

Chapter 8

Common Problems and Challenges

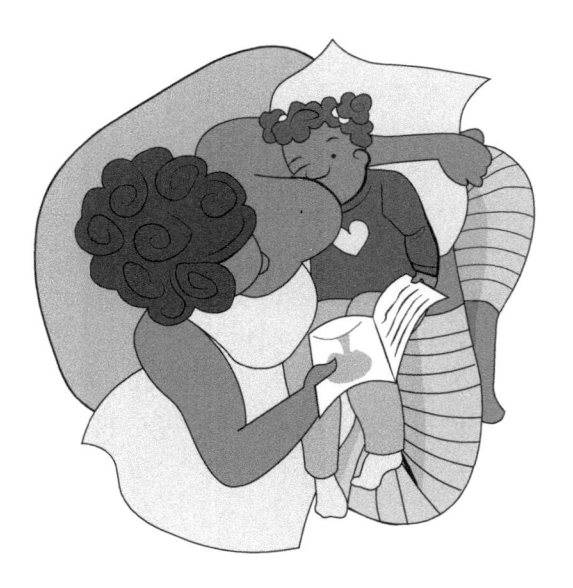

If a parent has been breastfeeding for six months, they have often overcome a number of hurdles. Many parents struggle to access sufficient and timely breastfeeding support, and finding someone who can devote time to your issue and is appropriately trained can be a challenge in itself. In the early days, discomfort is common and parents may need help with relieving engorgement, managing positioning and attachment issues. They may need support because they have concerns around insufficient milk supply (which may be perceived insufficient milk supply) or issues resulting from a lack of frequency of effective feeding. Lactation consultants who are busy supporting new parents may talk about tongue-tie, nipple infection, windiness or colic. We may support with insufficient weight gain or over-production. For most parents, by six months, worries are usually behind them. Breastfeeding feels established. Predictable patterns are developing. They know how things work, but of course it's not always plain sailing and problems can arise at any point in a breastfeeding experience even after several months without difficulties, or even after several years.

It is important to acknowledge that continuing to breastfeed can bring enormous challenges. Parents are so used to having to justify their breastfeeding relationship that it can sometimes feel disloyal to speak negatively about their experience. It feels as though they have signed up for some kind of charter where the normalization of breastfeeding older children requires them to focus on its 'benefits' and the positives. However, many parents are struggling and feeling the impact of their additional isolation. Dr Sally Dowling spoke to many parents breastfeeding older children in her research:

> Many of the women I spoke to for my research did not set out to breastfeed a toddler. They did not set out from pregnancy thinking that they were going to breastfeed an older child. Only one person I spoke to had made that decision in pregnancy. For most it was described as something that 'just happened'. Many of the women I spoke to found it really difficult, so although they were very clear that they felt it was the right thing to do, it didn't mean that they found it easy. They often found it very hard. This was about a combination of things. Sometimes it was about lack of sleep. They may have chosen to co-sleep but it did not mean that they found it easy. For some it was about combining work or maintaining relationships. And these women often have a real sense of determination. They start doing it,

> and over time they feel more and more it's the right thing to do. They learn more about it, perhaps get a community of women around them who are also doing it, and they become determined to carry on. Many women described a kind of 'bloody mindedness' that kept them going. The experience, for some, can be quite horrible. Some of the women I spoke to said that they struggled in their relationship and they were finding it impossible to think about how they could have another child because the one child they had was consuming them, all their time and energy, because of the way they had chosen to parent.
>
> ~ (Dr Sally Dowling)

Imagine you are a parent with sore nipples for the first time, breastfeeding a four-year-old. There may be few people in your life who are aware you are still breastfeeding. You may consciously have decided not to mention it to your family doctor or health visitor and now you need help. You may not feel able to visit a local support group that is very much newborn focused. If you have a four-year-old who breastfeeds regularly throughout the day and night, soreness can quickly escalate into something that impacts on your mental health as well as your physical health. What are some of the common concerns when breastfeeding older children?

As babies get older, they get heavier. Positioning and attachment will change. A parent who has been relying on the same positions used in early babyhood may find that gradually gravity starts to cause a problem. A seven-month-old baby may sink further into that breastfeeding pillow (that is less firm than it was seven months ago when it popped out of its packaging). Arms and hands may be struggling to support weight (especially if a parent is using a hand to support a head and neck of a baby in a cross-cradle hold). Positioning and attachment may be an issue at any age. We will ask questions about the shape of the nipple on exit. Is it flattened/ridged/looking like a new lipstick? Does it appear paler as if blood has been removed from the area? Does the parent finish a feed with an ache in their wrists and arms or back? Or a sense of relief that they can now relax? It may be time to discuss leaning back more and using what Nancy Mohrbacher terms 'natural breastfeeding'. Breastfeeding positions where parents sit upright are less common from birth than they once were as we are increasingly understanding the value of the baby being anchored and using positions that allow them to tap into their natural reflexes. Dr Suzanne Colson's work on what she describes as 'biological nurturing' and Mohrbacher's resources have transformed many breastfeeding experiences for parent and baby. (For information on Colson's work, see www.biologicalnurturing.com/pages/publications.html.) As Mohrbacher explains:

> In the commonly used cradle, cross-cradle, and football/rugby holds, mothers and babies must fight the effects of gravity to get babies to breast level and keep their fronts touching. If gaps form between them (which can happen easily with gravity pulling baby's body down and away), this disorients baby, which can lead to latching struggles. The pull of gravity makes it impossible for a newborn to use his inborn responses to get to his food source and feed. For baby, it is like trying to climb Mount Everest. Instead of mothers and babies working together as breastfeeding partners, mothers must do all of the work. Instead of being able to relax while baby helps, most mothers sit hunched over, tense, and struggling.
>
> To complicate things further, in these positions, gravity can transform the same inborn feeding responses that should be helping babies into barriers to breastfeeding. Head bobbing becomes head butting. Arm and leg movements meant to move babies to the breast become pushing and kicking. Mothers struggling to manage their babies' arms and legs in these upright breastfeeding holds have often told me: 'I don't think I have enough hands to breastfeed.' (Mohrbacher 2015)

This may all sound like a conversation relevant only to early breastfeeding. Surely once we've got to seven and eight months, this is all behind us? But in fact, parents who may have managed to get the more upright positions to work in the early days may find problems arising later on and conversations about reclined positions do start to become useful. Backs may only start to ache later on. Distractible babies may pull off and look around in positions where they are under the breast and being brought to the breast, but more cooperative in positions where they are more prone. It might be that flow is faster than a baby enjoys and a reclined position gives them more of a sense of control.

Babies' heads are bigger. In the early days, your baby may have rested naturally in a cradle-hold position and their chin neatly came to the breast and the nipple bobbed around their nose allowing a head tilt and an effective gape and mouthful of breast with an asymmetrical latch (more of a mouthful below the nipple). But it may be that as a baby's face has changed shape, they started to come beyond the breast a little more. That is to say that it was less 'nose to nipple' and more 'mouth to nipple' and eventually the head tilt may have shifted and the chin moved away from being buried in the breast and closer to pointing towards the nursling's chest. These changes happen slowly and imperceptibly.

The rugby hold/football hold may have been relied on in the early days, but if the cushions stay the same and the parent's position on the sofa doesn't change, where does the longer baby go? The length of their body starts to creep out in front of the breast, again leading to less chin contact, more latching above the nipple and the nipple potentially being pressed against the hard palate, rather than having the chance to be scooped back towards the soft palate.

Is a parent still using the same nursing chair? Where is the length of the baby now going? Are they still able to start 'nose to nipple'? This loss of the head tilt and the older baby smooshing into a breast nose-first is a common cause of later nipple pain. As the latch shifts and becomes less deep and effective, the nursling may start to compensate. They may suck harder in compensation, compress the nipple, pull on and off and behave

Common Problems and Challenges

in a fussier way at the breast. This could then cause further pain when the underlying issue was the shift in original positioning and attachment.

What else could be going on? Nipple compression can cause vasospasm when the removal of blood from the nipple under pressure can cause whitening. Vasospasm may also be caused by circulation issues such as Raynaud's syndrome – where blood vessels constrict in colder temperatures typically resulting in white fingertips and toes for those with paler skin (and sometimes other colour changes for those with darker skin). For a breastfeeding parent who gives birth in the spring, this may only start to become a significant cause of pain as the temperatures drop several months later.

Sarah Pett struggled with vasospasm:

> The first GP I saw about the vasospasm told me that I sounded like I'd spent too much time on the internet and said they'd look it up and then call me back in a week – an eternity for a new mother! I went back the next day with a printout of a medical journal article on vasospasm and treatment (which I could access because I worked for a university) and luckily the GP I saw then was sensitive and supportive. They agreed to prescribe me nifedipine, which didn't eliminate the pain but took the edge off just enough for me to persevere.
>
> ~ (Sarah Pett)

Keeping the area warm, perhaps having a hot water bottle or heat pack to apply once the feed is over, may also be helpful. There is also some evidence that vitamin B supplements may reduce attacks. If a parent describes vasospasm, the first step is to discuss nipple shaping and rule out nipple compression due to positioning and attachment.

For many families breastfeeding beyond the first six months, teeth come and go with minimal impact on breastfeeding. Come, as in they arrive after the first few months (typically between six and 12 months).

Go, as in they may even start to be lost as milk teeth fall out at around six years old alongside breastfeeding. The loss of milk teeth is often considered a natural marker for the end to breastfeeding. Some nurslings may find that palate changes that come with age at around the same time make it more challenging to maintain a seal on the breast and breastfeeding, certainly for nutritional purposes, fades away. In her article, 'A time to wean', Kathy Dettwyler describes the work of Holly Smith in examining the relationship between primate weaning age and arrival of first permanent molars. This connection was observed in 21 species of non-human primates and, if applied to humans, suggests our natural weaning age is around five and a half to six years old (Dettwyler 1995).

At the beginning of the arrival of teeth, some families are nervous. There is a fear that teeth may mean biting, but in fact, teeth aren't part of the mechanics of breastfeeding as it's in the baby's interests to keep them out of the way. The first teeth to erupt are usually the lower incisors which will be covered by an extended tongue during breastfeeding. Once the upper incisors emerge, there may be a period of re-adjustment but the breast is placed behind the upper teeth if the nursling's head is tilted in the optimum position. If the nursling is feeding with the chin closer down towards the chest, rather than away from the chest (a position that can sometimes develop as nurslings get older), that can mean the nose pressed into the breast and a greater chance of the teeth indenting and discomfort. If the emergence of teeth does bring pain, it's time to review positioning and attachment and reinforce the need for a large gape which scoops the breast towards the soft palate. We might talk to the nursling about using a 'big mouth' and 'head back' and encourage them to bring their chin to the breast first and the nipple starting around the nose. Older nurslings that have developed the habit of slurping the nipple in with a smaller gape are more likely to cause discomfort once teeth arrive. It cannot be under-estimated how much a nursling can be a partner in the process of adjustment. We can often explain what needs to change and why and they often get it and adapt.

That's not to say that biting never occurs. It can sometimes be

Common Problems and Challenges

more of an issue with younger babies who are using nothing but gum, perhaps clamping down as they fall asleep. With older babies it may be brief and experimental and it can be a shock. It is sometimes suggested that if a baby does bite, a parent should try not to react. A sudden loud reaction may even frighten and has been known to lead to a nursing strike. However, this is easier said than done. If a baby does bite, what is going on? Has anything recently changed? Some soft-spouted cups aimed at toddlers use valves which rely on a bite to release liquid. Could the introduction of a new cup have made a difference? Has teething started and might they appreciate the option to bite down on other things? Could there have recently been a reduction in milk flow (perhaps after a bout of mastitis) and the bite is flow protest? Sometimes flow protest may be in response to fast and overwhelming flow instead.

It can be worth reviewing feeding patterns overall. Has the parent/baby partnership historically been feeding using typical intervals in the day? Has responsive feeding naturally slid into a more predictable schedule which is less about cues and more about a system that seems to work? Perhaps the baby is ready for longer intervals? It may be that solids intake has increased and a bite is the only way that a message of 'For goodness sake, I don't want milk now' can be conveyed. It may be that the baby is ready for a feed that has a shorter duration. In the early months of breastfeeding, it is unfortunately still drilled into many parents that a successful feed must be X number of minutes long. If this magic X number is not reached (and X could be anything from 10 to 40 minutes depending on who you speak to), the baby may not reach sufficient fatty milk. The term 'hindmilk' is still sometimes used in these conversations – a term that few lactation specialists employ as it gives the misleading impression there are different kinds of breastmilk. In reality, some feeds may start with a high proportion of fattier milk than others. In some breasts, depending on the number of milk ducts, or the force of the milk ejection reflex or the fullness of the milk storage areas, the fat content of a feed will start to rise within moments. It may take three minutes or 13 minutes for the same proportion of fatty milk to be reached. The UNICEF UK Baby Friendly Initiative assessment sheets, used by health professionals from birth, talk of a newborn feed being around five to 40 minutes in length (UNICEF UK Baby Friendly Initiative 2018). A newborn feeding successfully and putting on weight well may only feed for five minutes at a time. However, this message has still not reached even the parents of older babies who may still be battling to get to a magic X but now with a child who is increasingly efficient at the breast and not remotely interested in feeding for a moment longer than is necessary. A bite may again be the way to communicate 'I'm done!' or 'Will you PLEASE stop trying to reattach me because you think I should be feeding for three more minutes because your app tells you I should be!'

When a bite does happen, after the moments of ouch, and the moments of analysis, we want to talk to parents about moist wound healing and keeping any damaged skin clean by washing with mild soap and water to reduce the risk of infection. A bite cannot easily happen if a baby is actively swallowing as the tongue is extended. For a bite to occur, the tongue is retracted and that will usually be signalled by a shift in the jaw and often what parents describe as a 'twinkle in the eye'. We can encourage parents to look out for that jaw shift and have a little finger poised to break the vacuum and detach. Often, once a baby realizes that a bite means detachment, and even being placed on the floor, it quickly loses its appeal. In the moment of a sudden bite, it might be instinctive to pull a baby off, but actually, bringing a baby into the breast may be more useful. When a baby is smooshed into the breast and their breathing is restricted, it means no danger for them but they will immediately detach and pull back. A firm 'no' may be appropriate, depending on the age of the baby, and sometimes it just makes the parent feel better.

A parent that has been bitten may be afraid but they can be reassured that biting is rare and is preventable. It goes without saying that messages that this means a natural ending to breastfeeding are unhelpful and likely to cause more upset at an emotional time. It is a common trope to associate teeth and biting with breastfeeding an older child.

Common Problems and Challenges

The 'horror' some feel around continued breastfeeding and their natural instinct to wince can be meshed with a reference to breastfeeding an older child with teeth. There may be a 'How could you...' which pretends the issue is teeth on breast but really the discomfort goes further. In reality, for almost all parents who breastfeed an older child, even up to the emergence of permanent teeth, there is rarely a problem. When problems do occur, they are often temporary and fixable. Nurslings want to transfer milk effectively and they want nursing sessions to be welcome for everyone and relaxing.

> Jacob also had a long biting episode at nine months old which coincided with me re-starting my periods. It was so bad I bled after most feeds and dreaded each feed. I thought I had reached the end of our breastfeeding journey and cried a lot about this as I have enjoyed it so much and felt I wouldn't be able to mother him the same without this. My health visitor encouraged me to speak to the national breastfeeding support line before I gave in, and they gave me useful tips which enabled me to continue to feed. Since [then] we have had no biting and Jacob continues to enjoy feeding and has learnt to baby sign for milk and laughs when he does so. Breastfeeding is still his safe, warm space.
>
> ~ (Anna)
>
> My second daughter Daisy (now 14 months) got teeth quite early (at five months) and by 14 months has almost all of them. She has always bitten me when she is teething and it is so painful and always a shock! She has drawn blood a couple of times too which I found quite upsetting. I know the advice is to try to not react and just unlatch them, or to try to anticipate when the bite might occur and take them off before that happens. This was hard with Daisy as she would often look at me and smile as she took a bite! I changed tack and would take her off and say, 'Off', and say, 'We use gentle teeth, no

biting, that hurts Mummy.' I put her back on if she asks for more milk, but sometimes if she continues to bite me, I say she can have more later and put her down. One day, when she was about nine months old, she was holding one of the dummies whilst she was feeding (she doesn't really use a dummy, but she does play with them sometimes) and she came off and bit the dummy instead of my nipple! I was so touched and found it amazing that she had come up with her own solution to this problem! So now if she is teething or she is in a biting phase, I try to make sure we have one of the dummies or a teething toy for her to bite instead of me when she is feeding and this has worked really well so far!

~ *(Holly)*

Why else might a parent be experiencing nipple pain? With the advent of teething, there can be a change in saliva production. Some state that saliva is more 'acidic' but there appears to be little evidence for this. However, it may be that increased saliva production could cause more nipple sensitivity, just as it may cause a baby to have a cheek or chin rash. An older baby may also have particles of solid food in their mouth which parental skin may react to. There may also be other reasons for an allergic reaction such as a change in nipple cream, soap or detergent. Perhaps where previously a nipple was protected by a breast pad, now it is coming directly into contact with fabric as leaking has stopped.

Nipple sensitivity may also be a result of hormonal changes including a phase of the menstrual cycle or a subsequent pregnancy as we'll discuss more in Chapter 9, which covers conception, pregnancy and tandem feeding. The return of the menstrual period will affect parents in different ways. It may also come at very different times. Some exclusively breastfeeding parents will see a return of a menstrual cycle after as early as four to six weeks. This can be shocking to some, and some fear it means an end to breastfeeding, but breastfeeding can successfully continue alongside a full menstrual cycle for years. Others may take 12 to 18 months for a period to return. In terms of challenges the menstrual cycle can bring, some parents do report an increase in their nursling's fussiness for a few days during their cycle, beginning usually just prior to the onset of bleeding. It's possible that hormonal changes are causing a slight supply reduction and potentially that the taste of the milk may change. It may also be that nipples are more tender, or the parent may experience some aversion, for short periods. Some report that symptoms are worse prior to a first period, but once a cycle is more established, they become easier to manage. Calcium and magnesium supplements are sometimes recommended to reduce symptoms. *The Womanly Art of Breastfeeding*, published by La Leche League, states: 'A daily dose of 500–1,000 mg of a calcium and magnesium supplement from the middle of your cycle through the first three days of your period may help minimize any drop in supply' (Wiessinger, West and Pitman 2010, p.193).

There is no strong evidence to support this but it is an intervention we can place in the category of 'unlikely to do harm', and at the very least, it may be a valuable placebo if a parent is worried. As Nancy Mohrbacher points out, 'for the vast majority of parents, milk production is a hardy process' (Mohrbacher 2020) and we need to be careful not to send messages that normal biological processes mean fragility to breastfeeding. When we live in a society where perceptions of low milk supply are common, without foundation, we need to be careful not to exaggerate the impact of the return of the menstrual cycle. It may be that someone's period has returned because they have been removing milk less frequently in recent weeks and that is the cause of any noticeable decrease, rather than the period itself.

Infections on the nipple may also be a cause of nipple pain. It may be easier to distinguish an infection with a more experienced breastfeeding parent as after a period of pain-free breastfeeding, a sudden change, particularly accompanied by a change in nipple appearance, is less likely to be confused with positioning and attachment challenges. Thrush on the nipple may be a cause of pain, especially after a course of antibiotics for either nursling or parent. Parents who have paler skin tones may notice nipples appear pinker than usual. Parents with darker skin tones may notice a loss of pigment on the areola. Parents may report a scaliness on the nipple and increased sensitivity. Symptoms will quickly transfer to both sides and miconazole oral gel is the recommended treatment for the nursling and the cream for the parent. Some practitioners emphasize the need for a swab to be taken to identify thrush as the culprit.

If only one nipple is painful after several days, especially if it's accompanied by a yellow crustiness, a bacterial infection should be considered with topical ointment given. Parents can also be advised to wash with mild soap and water first to break down any bacterial biofilm and reduce the risk of mastitis, then apply a topical antibiotic cream (Walker 2013). A staph aureus infection may also present as impetigo on the nipple, with crusty sores. Impetigo on the nipple is unlikely to be a common issue when a parent is breastfeeding a baby, but more of a consideration once a nursling is 18 months and over. There may be an assumption that breastfeeding can easily be suspended as impetigo is highly infectious, but of course, as we have discussed, it is rarely 'easy' when it comes to temporarily suspending breastfeeding with an older nursling and the dyad is likely to want to continue breastfeeding alongside treatment.

Older nurslings may also present with cold sores (herpes simplex). If the family are tandem feeding and breastfeeding a young baby under three weeks, it is important to note that cold sores can be dangerous and even fatal for newborns (NHS 2018b). If one breast is without cold sore lesions, it may be possible for one breast to be used for feeding the baby but it is important the baby does not come into contact with lesions, and breastfeeding for the toddler may need to be paused. If the only nursling is an older child, there is a strong argument for continuing to breastfeed as normal as the contagious period has already started one or two days before the lesions become visible.

Other viruses such as hand, foot and mouth disease, chicken pox and fifth disease are not a reason to stop breastfeeding, although a pregnant parent should consult with their doctor. A child with hand, foot and mouth disease may be particularly troubled with sores in their mouth but there is research to suggest breastfeeding can reduce symptoms. Other skin conditions on the nipple such as eczema and psoriasis should be treatable without an assumption that breastfeeding should end.

Blebs or milk blisters are a result of a duct-opening becoming blocked at the surface of the nipple. This may be because an older nursling's 'nose first' positioning style causes the nipple to rub against the hard palate or insufficient gaping may mean tongue abrasion against the nipple. A change in positioning style may be a long-term solution, but in the short term, hot compresses, massage with warm olive oil, Epsom salt soaks and gently and hygienically breaking the skin over the bleb may help.

Blocked ducts deeper in the breast can happen at any point in a breastfeeding experience. When nurslings are older, risks may be greater during the weaning process. Milk stasis can occur when milk storage areas are at full capacity without regular effective milk removal and milk starts to leak into tissue where it will be treated as a foreign body. The link with positioning and attachment issues should be reviewed. When a toddler's hand is pressed into the breast, a toddler's latch is shallow or 'gymnurstics' means pulling and playing at the breast, the risk of blocked ducts increases.

The risk of mastitis is greater in the first three months but it can occur at any time. If a parent has nipple damage, their risk will be higher. During the weaning process, they should also be vigilant for signs of unresolved blocked ducts.

Nursing strikes can happen at any point in a breastfeeding career. However, as we approach the second half of the first year, there are pinch points. From as early as four months, babies may start to see breastfeeding as an annoyance taking them away from a world that appears increasingly interesting. Daytime breastfeeds can be more of a battle or an ongoing distraction game. A six- or seven-month-old baby may breastfeed for short periods in the day or reverse cycle, and compensate with more feeding at night. They may appear very reluctant to come to the breast in the day and a parent may feel as though they are battling to make feeds happen. This may feel very much like a nursing strike although it is a common phase, often accompanied by shorter breastfeeds when breastfeeding does happen.

A nine- or ten-month-old may strike for a variety of reasons. As mentioned previously, a reaction to a biting episode may be the trigger. A parent's yelp of surprise may mean a baby is nervous to return to the breast but this can be framed as a baby worried about hurting someone he cares about rather than a rejection. A nursling may have other health issues such as an ear infection or sore throat or discomfort from teething. A parent may feel they have to identify 'the reason', but it may never be known. Most practitioners agree that a strike under 12 months should not be confused with self-weaning. However, it may not be helpful to stick to a strict definition of what constitutes self-weaning in the face of a family who chooses to define it as such. The common understanding is that self-weaning is a gradual process and it rarely occurs under 18 months. If a family was not anticipating the end of breastfeeding and their goals were not to wean imminently, there is no reason to believe a strike has to be the end. Nursing strikes may last as long as seven to ten days. A parent needs to be supported to protect their milk supply and attempt the impossible to 'stay relaxed' when they may feel as though they are at risk of suddenly losing something precious. It feels like rejection at the most fundamental level even if a parent's logical brain knows that isn't true.

> 'She had a nursing strike at around one year. I found it incredibly upsetting, and I think it was at this point that I realized how important continuing breastfeeding really was to me.'
>
> ~ (Naomi)

A nursing strike may end with sleepy feeding or reclined relaxed feeding. A sleepy baby may accept the breast and resume feeding before their conscious brain has even noticed that's what they are doing. Parents should be supported to 'offer' the breast without 'pushing' the breast. Having a bath together, hanging out skin-to-skin or offering other distractions (movement, singing) may help. In very rare cases, strikes may extend beyond what feels comfortable and parents may choose to consider it the end of breastfeeding for their own mental health as much as anything. They may not feel comfortable living with a longer period of uncertainty and the constant tension of wondering when the strike is going to end and wish to take control. That isn't to say that they didn't wish for breastfeeding to continue but that they decided to draw a line under the expectation that it will end imminently. In this situation, breastfeeding grief and trauma is a natural response and a parent will need additional emotional support.

Many of us live in a society where perceived insufficient milk (PIM) supply is a common problem. Lisa Gatti reports that 'PIM is often reported as the most common problem that women experience with breastfeeding' (Gatti 2008). It is more easily identified as an issue in the early weeks and months when parents may be unfamiliar with normal infant behaviour and the natural patterns of responsive feeding, cluster feeding and the baby's desire for closeness. They may also be confused by breast changes such as reduced engorgement, reduced sensation from the milk ejection reflex ('letdown reflex') and increased breast softness. When once parents could feel which breast to feed more next, the letdown reflex was a noticeable tingle and leaking was constant, things have changed. Too often, these natural changes are interpreted as a reduction in milk supply. Pumping output may also decrease as the body becomes more efficient at storing and making milk to meet baby's needs or the pump itself may be ready for a service and replacement parts after several months of usage. We would expect feeds to be getting shorter, but after months of believing 'more minutes = good' that can be a hard adjustment. If a parent after six months is still using an app that counts the minutes of a feed, it's important to have conversations that explain how shorter feeds are the expectation as babies get older and do not necessarily lead to a smaller intake. It can be useful to help them to reflect on when it's time to move away from the app, and the positives and negatives of measuring breastfeeds when breastfeeding is so much more than a milk delivery system.

You might imagine that a lack of confidence in milk supply fades as we pass the six-month mark but there is no magic age at which parents are no longer impacted. As babies start to sleep for longer intervals at night, parents may become nervous that their milk supply will reduce and should be reassured that some engorgement and some adjustment to their milk supply is normal and this does not mean an insufficiency of milk. Starting solids can be another source of anxiety. Parents, especially those who may have had early battles with weight gain and phasing out supplements, may worry that their baby will be less interested in the breast or may not have the right balance between solids intake and breastmilk. I have known some parents to find the introduction of solid food emotional as it can feel like a loss and the end of an era, rather than always something 'exciting' that they 'must be looking forward to'. It can also trigger anxiety that milk intake will fall too rapidly and supply will be impacted.

In some cases, the concerns around milk supply may have some foundation. It may be that the use of supplements or sleeping training or a desire for more structure in the day (and the introduction of some sort of feeding schedule) has had a negative impact on milk production. It may also be that a parent has started to take hormonal contraception for the first time after six months of the lactational amenorrhoea method (LAM) of birth control. This method of birth control can be 98–99% effective in preventing pregnancy provided a baby is under six months, exclusively and responsively breastfeeding and periods have not returned. This would mean breastfeeding is unrestricted and both night and day. Some sources suggest a baby needs to feed at least every four hours in the day and at least every six hours at night. Going longer than that, including if the parent is expressing, may not be enough to suppress ovulation (Family Planning Association 2017; Planned Parenthood 2021). Once one of these conditions is no longer met, parents may turn to hormonal contraception. From six months, all forms of hormonal contraception are considered compatible with breastfeeding. However, as Wendy Jones, the specialist pharmacist with the UK's Breastfeeding Network, points out: 'Breastfeeding advocates worldwide seem to be aware of anecdotal reports of lowered, lost milk supply but these reports do not appear to have been published leading to variance with academic researchers' (Jones 2021).

If a parent breastfeeding successfully appears to notice issues with their milk supply shortly after starting hormonal contraception, many would make the connection that it should be at least considered that the contraception could be responsible. It may be wise to start with oral progestin (progesterone)-only pills to assess impact before moving to injectable contraception or long-acting methods that cannot be reversed. It may also be that a parent who feels supply decreasing unexpectedly is pregnant, and this may be possible even before the return of their period if the first egg is 'caught'.

If a baby's fussiness is a cause for concern, and weight gain appears to be slowing beyond what can be normal developmental ups and downs, parents can be reassured that milk production can be increased at any age with efficient milk removal and increased stimulation. It may be that positioning and attachment need a review and a small tweak can start to turn things around as feeds become more effective.

Parents who have been breastfeeding for longer may be influenced by peers to consider herbal galactagogues or lactation cookies and this requires caution. Even if we consider these harmless placebos, do we really want a placebo that normalizes perceptions of low milk supply? Or one that may contain ingredients that are expensive and potentially harmful to parents with certain health conditions? If they are to be used, it should at the very least be alongside accurate information and an investigation as to what the underlying causes may be.

Concerns around milk supply may also include over-supply. This is particularly a concern for parents in the first few weeks and usually supply has regulated by the third and fourth months. Sometimes it may feel like an ongoing battle. A parent breastfeeding an older child should be supported to regulate supply and should feel more confident to do so. There are some concerns that frequent use of silicone milk 'catchers', that may exert some negative pressure on the breast and do more than simply catch a milk ejection reflex, could be contributing to over-production. Weaning may be a nerve-wracking time as it may lead to a greater risk of discomfort or blocked ducts. Cold compresses, use of green cabbage leaf compresses and the use of sage may be considered. Kelly Bonyata, IBCLC, reports: 'To use dried sage (Salvia officinalis) for reducing milk supply, take 1/4 teaspoon of sage 3 x per day for 1–3 days' (Bonyata 2018a).

If you speak to a family who is breastfeeding a toddler or older child, one of the advantages often cited is the fact that when a child is unwell and off their food, being able to offer milk is a huge relief. If a child is congested, they may need help being able to feed and breathe comfortably. That might include the use of saline drops or feeding in a steamy bathroom. If a child has vomiting or diarrhoea, there can sometimes be confusion, especially if health professionals supporting the family are not used to meeting older nurslings. If a child is able to have anything orally, breastmilk is a sound first choice. I doubt anyone reading this needs reminding that breastmilk is not a 'dairy product'. There is no logic in replacing breastmilk, nature's ultimate rehydrating solution, with a powdered rehydrating solution such as Pedialyte unless it is absolutely necessary. Breastmilk is 88% water, is easily digestible and contains antibodies. If a health professional does appear to be advocating the cessation of breastfeeding, which also provides comfort during a stressful time, they will need to be able to provide some convincing evidence. Oral rehydration therapy may be a helpful tool if breastfeeding is not happening frequently or sufficiently, but breastfeeding is a first choice. If a child is reluctant to nurse, they may also prefer to be spoon-fed, syringe-fed or lick a frozen breastmilk ice lolly. If a child has diarrhoea, it may take a while for their stools to return to normal as secondary lactose intolerance may be a temporary effect of an infection. Continuing breastmilk and not confusing the symptoms for an allergy or intolerance to breastmilk is the recommendation of health professionals familiar with children who are breastfeeding (Newman 2017).

When a child is very unwell, it's not always as simple as 'support exclusive breastfeeding at all costs'. There can be complex issues. Lyndsey Hookway IBCLC, is passionate about supporting medically complex infants and children who are breastfeeding. She offers training to fellow medical professionals as well as highlighting the importance of peer support through her 'Breastfeeding the Brave' Facebook group for families. Her PhD is specifically focused on supporting medically complex infants and children in the paediatric setting.

Hookway outlines the issues:

> Breastfeeding medically complex children is an entirely different challenge to establishing breastfeeding or troubleshooting problems with healthy infants and children. Very sick children often have huge challenges and obstacles to overcome. However, one of the main obstacles is that the support in the paediatric setting is severely lacking. With well-established guidelines, audit procedures and infant feeding specialist roles in neo-natology, community and maternity services, paediatrics so far feels like the forgotten arm of breastfeeding support (Hookway, Lewis and Brown 2021).
>
> The paediatric medical and nursing team are wonderful at supporting critically, seriously and terminally ill children, but have limited or no experience in supporting breastfeeding, or maintaining lactation. Breastfeeding counsellors, peer supporters and IBCLCs are excellent at supporting breastfeeding in many difficult circumstances, but may not have encountered many really sick children, especially in the in-patient setting.
>
> What we need is for paediatric professionals and lactation professionals to meet in the middle (Hookway 2020). If professionals can

work together to find creative solutions, the outcomes for families would be much more positive.

As much as we promote exclusive breastfeeding, sometimes there are babies who cannot be exclusively breastfed, for example babies with certain metabolic conditions. We need to look at the bigger picture beyond just prioritizing breastfeeding. Some of this is about empowering parents but it's also about change coming from within structures and organizations. Support for breastfeeding needs to come from higher up. This needs to be about grassroots training because at the moment breastfeeding isn't part of the standard training for lots of health professionals and many universities don't have to teach it. NMC education standards cover complex feeding situations but not normal oral feeding. (NMC is the Nursing and Midwifery Council – the nursing and midwifery regulator for England, Wales, Scotland and Northern Ireland.)

A lot of the literature around breastfeeding sick kids relates to some really specific conditions. Any paediatric nurse on the paediatric ward who's under pressure doesn't have time to look for the Down syndrome breastfeeding guideline or the sickle cell guideline or the cystic fibrosis guideline. What we need is a paediatric feeding assessment tool for all babies on admission to the ward which would pull out any feeding issues we need to look at. Some of the common problems may include low tone, an inability to form a safe seal, suck/swallow/breathe sequencing, difficulty positioning the child at the breast around lines, transitioning from intubation, tube feeding back to oral feeding, high caloric needs or reduced volume tolerance. Whether a child has low tone because of cerebral palsy or Down syndrome, you could just then follow guidelines around low tone and utilize specific strategies that manage that clinical problem.

We also need to have an identified paediatric feeding team. At the moment, there is a neo-natal infant feeding team and a maternity infant feeding team but they are unlikely to be able to support a family in paediatrics because there may not be funding, or time. It may also be outside of their skillset, depending on their experience and training. After all, supporting a parent to express for their preterm baby, and then transition to direct breastfeeding when the infant is ready, is a very different challenge from supporting a child after open-heart surgery, or during cancer treatment. So we've got paediatrics slipping through the gap in the middle.

Some people breastfeeding older children might have continued to breastfeed through their child's illness anyway. Perhaps they do this because they are parents who value natural-term weaning or it might be that they continued for longer because of the immunological benefits. When I have told people that I breastfed my youngest child until she was five years and nine months, I have often then suffixed that with: 'I probably wouldn't have continued so long if she hadn't been diagnosed with cancer. I breastfed her through all of her chemo.' People often respond by saying, 'Well, that's understandable', as if it wouldn't be understandable if she had an intact immune system. I've stopped doing that of late. Rather than saying I did it because of that, I say I did it as well as that.

Another challenge that a family may face is parental separation. This can happen when a child is any age, or even during pregnancy, but there may be unique considerations if we are talking about a family where an older child is breastfeeding. When we live in a society where breastfeeding beyond babyhood is not always understood, let alone valued, it is unlikely that a court system will have a full appreciation of the role of breastfeeding in a family's life. Ideally decisions about access and visitation will be reached between parents and sometimes with the help of a mediator. Continuing to breastfeed is not a barrier for a child to spend time with another parent. Breastfeeding parents regularly work night shifts, work away from home or even travel for work. However, the relationship between a child and their primary caregiver can also not be dismissed as not worthy of prioritizing during discussions. If an older child is breastfeeding, this is not a conversation about access to milk but access to an adult they have a secure attachment to, at a time in life when secure attachments are paramount. It is a conversation that is about far more than milk delivery but one about trust, security and healthy attachment. Both parents will ideally be prioritizing the welfare of their child which includes facilitating the relationship with their co-parent, which benefits their child's physical and mental health and enables them to trust both parents in the long term. A child's secure attachment to a breastfeeding parent at night needs to be considered when reviewing parenting arrangements for overnight stays. It is logical that the move to overnight stays away from the breastfeeding parent happens gently and with both parents in cooperation. If both parties feel comfortable doing so, it may even be that a breastfeeding parent visits at bedtime for a final breastfeed and conveys the message that the other residence is a place where they also feel safe and comfortable. A non-breastfeeding parent may visit the other parent's home to assist with bedtime after a day of contact. There are as many variations as there are families. This is time to get creative. It may be that the child's location initially stays constant and parents take turns to spend time with the child. As a child gets older, locations may vary more easily. Of course, this may be too challenging depending on the relationship between the parents, but it is likely that the child's best interests will be served by parents being willing to make some sort of sacrifice. That might mean spending time with someone you would prefer not to spend time with or being more patient about the move to overnight stays than you might like.

What is not appropriate, and is contrary to the rights of both children and parents, is a requirement that breastfeeding an older child ends to facilitate custody arrangements. This is simply missing the point and contrary to the child's human rights. The end of breastfeeding does not remove the fact that the child has a secure attachment to the breastfeeding parent and it is THIS that needs to be supported while also ensuring the child's relationship with their other parent can flourish. If anyone is directed to end breastfeeding a letter written by Kathy Dettwyler, available online, may be useful to share with a court. She states:

It is quite feasible for divorced parents to work out shared custody or visitation arrangements that allow the father to have ample time with his child while not sacrificing the breastfeeding relationship the child has with its mother. There is no reason why the child cannot have close relationships with both parents, and other stakeholders (grandparents, aunts and uncles, and so on) including spending substantial amounts of time with both mother and father, without weaning having to take place before the child is ready. (Dettwyler 2015)

When a parent is breastfeeding an older child, it may have been some time since they last expressed milk and they may be worried about the impact on their health or their milk supply if they spend time away from their child. After a longer breastfeeding journey, breasts are usually more flexible in coping with longer intervals and milk supply is less sensitive. It is also likely that expressing and hand expressing will be easier when the breasts are fuller or when using techniques like massaging and hand expressing in a bath or shower. If a child is older than eight or nine months, and is able to eat solids and drink water, it is likely that they will not need access to other milk during daytime visits with the non-breastfeeding parent. There is no need to introduce formula milk if it is not the choice of both parents.

There is another challenge when it comes to breastfeeding older children that we have yet to address. There are older babies and older children who may latch for the first time beyond six months. In some cases, we may be talking about nursing dyads who had been previously dealing with medical complications preventing initial latching. In most cases, we will be talking about adoptive children and future nurslings joining a family for the first time. This situation will require skill and patience and an understanding of the fact breastfeeding is an emotional connection and far more than a food delivery system. Some future nurslings will require a step-by-step transition from a world where perhaps bottle-feeding was functional and lacked intimacy to the world of breastfeeding. There may also be historical trauma or other complications. For those professionals who lack experience supporting in this area, the first message is that it is absolutely possible for a child to latch and breastfeed for the very first time after many months and even beyond a year. Alyssa Schnell is a lactation consultant in the USA who specializes in this area, and her book *Breastfeeding Without Birthing* is a valuable resource (Schnell 2013). Families will define their own goals. For some, the focus may never be on nutrition but on all the other experiences a connection at the breast can provide. For a Muslim adopting family, it may be important that a child coming into the family breastfeeds so that the child becomes a mahram (a full family member, unmarriageable kin, someone who does not require covering in front of). A transition to breastfeeding can take time, requiring making a bottle more like a breastfeeding experience or even making a breastfeeding experience more like a bottle experience, or it may happen unexpectedly and suddenly at a child's request.

For parents

Positioning and attachment issues can arise at any point in a breastfeeding experience. You may think sore nipples are behind you but they may be directly in front of you even if your nursling is several years old. Sometimes the situation may have changed so slowly and gradually that you may not have been consciously aware of how things shifted.

If your latch is working, you are not in pain and your nursling is getting milk effectively, don't feel you have to change things because you aren't 'following the rules'. A latch of an older child may not look like the latching babies in the textbooks and that can be OK. However, if you are struggling, a tweak may make all the difference.

Here are a few of my favourite tweak considerations:

1) When we take a drink from a glass of water, notice how we tip our heads back and our chins come away from our chest. When we try to

take a drink with our chin pointing down towards our chest – not so easy. So, we need to ensure our nursling is in a position where they can lift their chin away from their chest. This is one of the leading causes for a painful latch with an older nursling. We talk about 'nose to nipple' because that's encouraging the baby to reach towards the nipple with their head tilted back. As they have grown, they are often gradually less 'nose to nipple' at the start of the feed and more 'mouth on first'. They may be looking into the breast, rather than looking past it. If you are using a cradle hold or a cross-cradle hold, that means you might need to have them further away from the feeding breast's armpit and slid more across towards the non-feeding breast. As they have got longer and bigger, this is likely to mean the centre of gravity moves further across your body. Their ear will not be resting on the same place as it was when they were a small baby. If you are using a rugby hold, it's important the nursling isn't too far forward so they end up curling around the breast with their chin hunched towards their chest. You may need to sit further forward on your chair, or change where you are sitting, to give your nursling space to be behind you. With an older child, it can be helpful to make them a conscious partner in the process and talk about 'head back and chin first' and 'big mouth'.

2) Beware the slurp. As babies get older, we have less control over how they approach the breast. They may jump on with a nipple slurp and use suction to draw the nipple inside their mouth. It may not matter much initially. It seems to work and it's not particularly uncomfortable for you. However, once upper incisor teeth are on the scene, this may come back to bite you (literally), so try and maintain the connection with 'big mouth' and the tongue and chin touching the breast first (to scoop breast tissue back into the mouth). Using lips to suck the nipple into the mouth is likely to mean a shallower latch with greater chance of the nipple rubbing against the hard palate and a tongue which isn't extended over the gum ridge – also exposing the breast to the lower incisors.

3) Beware cushions. Are you using the same cushions and the same chair you were using when your baby was smaller? It may be time for a change. You may find that you are having to lift your breast up from its natural position to meet your nursling's mouth which is now several centimetres higher than it once was. If you are having to accommodate your body to allow for the cushion, it may be time to abandon it altogether. What often works even better is no pillow at all and leaning back a bit. Check out Nancy Mohrbacher's resources on natural breastfeeding and her YouTube channel (see www.nancymohrbacher.com which includes a link to her YouTube channel). Even if you've never used a reclined position before, it's never too late to introduce the concept.

4) Make space for your nursling. Connected to a review of cushions is a review of where their torso is now fitting. If you've been using an upright position or a koala position, you may find that your nursling's head creeps gradually higher until they are no longer looking up at the breast with their chin away from their chest. In some cases, I've seen older toddlers sitting upright on laps coming down onto the breast from above. There's not much chance of tongue contact on the breast in that position. It can feel scary to abandon something that is familiar but it may be time for a re-think. You may still be able to use the koala hold but in a reclined position which means they start further down your body. A familiar nursing chair may no longer fit and you may have discovered your nursling's head shifting further and further around the breast to accommodate the lower end of their body.

5) A nursling needs to be close to the breast, and as an older baby or toddler wears more clothes, clothing may be bunching up between you and pushing their face away from the breast. Just a few millimetres may shallow the latch enough for it to become more uncomfortable. Also watch out for nursling arms. An arm pinned between you is chunkier and thicker than it once was!

Common Problems and Challenges

6) What's the bottom cheek doing? Get someone to check that the bottom cheek is touching the breast too. Sometimes as babies get bigger and heads get bigger, the bottom cheek starts to drift and may even be several centimetres away from the breast, causing a shallower latch on the underside. If a nursling is upright, they may twist their face from the breast to get a look at the room and one cheek comes away from the breast. This may not be a problem for you, but if you are uncomfortable, it may need adjusting. Can you place something else in their line of sight that might hold their attention such as a window or nursing necklace? With much older nurslings, you can simply explain that you find it uncomfortable.

7) Are the ear, shoulder and hip in alignment? Get that glass of water again. Twist your neck and try to take a drink. It's hard! And if what you were drinking was gradually getting thicker and fattier, again, you're likely to be taking in air and giving up sooner than you might. Baby can't lie on their back and twist their neck towards you to come to the breast, however much they would want to try. We want the ear and shoulder and hip to all be pointing in the same direction. Even a baby with a twisted torso when the twist is around the hips can run into problems. As the world gets more interesting, you may find babies want to turn away and be able to look at things and start to get more twisty. If it doesn't hurt and it seems to be working for everyone, that's not a problem. But it is a problem if you are in pain.

8) Don't make your baby eat cotton. Breastfeeding clothes can assume we're all the same but not all nipples are in the same place and not all breasts fall in the same way. If you find them a faff – as you pull open a teeny slit to find your nipple hidden in there somewhere – I'm pretty sure your nursling does too. If they ping back so the baby's nose and cheek comes back into contact with fabric again, maybe re-think. I've even seen nurslings with fabric in their mouths with a look of resignation that says, 'This is the best I'm going to get.' Cheap vest tops you can pull out of the way are very sensible. You can layer

more than one so different bits are covered. And a bulldog clip or hair clip is useful for securing fabric (not your chin holding your clothing and preventing it from flopping down onto baby's face). Your baby's mouth has got bigger, so a breastfeeding bra or top that worked in the early days may not fit their gaping mouth now.

9) Maybe your baby just doesn't want to feed. If their latch is shallow and fussy, if they are pulling off and slurping and bouncing around (the term 'gymnurstics' is sometimes used), it may not be the time to feed. An uncomfortable latch can be connected to a lack of motivation. Your nursling may be saying that they are not interested in feeding right now. That can be scary, particularly when you are used to feeds being no longer than three or four hours apart, but waiting may be positive. It may mean a nursling who is happy to get down to business and wants the most efficient latch possible to get the milk they want as effectively as possible. It may also be that they are ready for a shorter feed. Feeds don't have to last a certain amount of time for the nursling to reach the high-fat-content milk and we don't need to push them to stay on longer than they want to. The idea that the fat won't arrive for five or ten or 15 minutes isn't evidence-based information. One fat molecule may break away immediately. And its friends will gradually find their way over the next few minutes. The proportion of fat will increase gradually and steadily. There is no 'foremilk' or 'hindmilk'. There is just milk that gradually changes. And first milk that was lower in fat but rich in carbohydrates is not worth less. Your nursling may want to feed for just four or five minutes to meet their needs and that can be OK. If you are noticing that subsequent latches are more uncomfortable, they could just be saying, 'No thanks.'

10) Do you have a baby who battles breastfeeds in the day? The world is too interesting and they would much prefer to play or look around (sometimes taking your nipple with them). Some parents try and create a distraction-free environment for daytime feeds. This might

include blacking out a room or ensuring everything is as quiet as possible. However, this isn't always realistic, particularly if you are caring for other children. Sometimes it's preferable to go the other way and make breastfeeding stimulating. Don't use a boring old cradle hold but try an upright koala hold. Bounce on a birthing ball. Fiddle with their hand or wave their arm around while you make a funny noise. Sit by a window so their line of sight on the breast is something interesting. Wear some chunky jewellery or get a nursing necklace. Sometimes nurslings will latch on while being half-distracted, and feed before they have noticed that's what they are doing. However, if your baby is still resisting feeding, and they otherwise seem well, trust that they will let you know when they are ready. It may be disconcerting when you are used to more frequent feeding but patterns change and nurslings will usually be OK.

However old your nursling is, it is never too late to reach out for help from a peer supporter, breastfeeding counsellor or lactation consultant if you are worried.

Chapter 9

Getting Pregnant Again

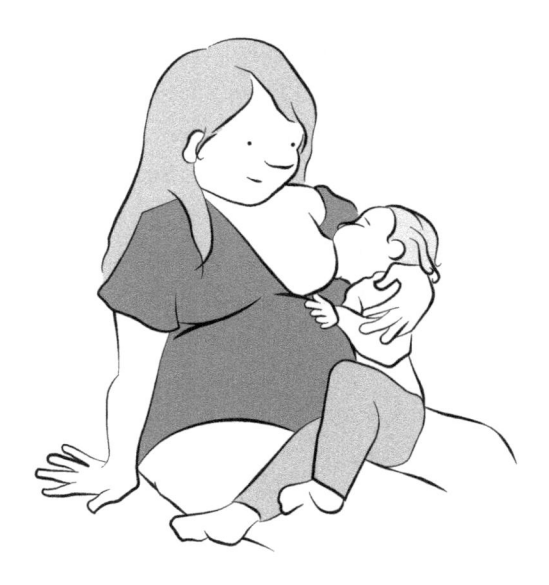

One of the areas where parents struggle most against the 'myth-monster' is the world of continuing to breastfeed during a subsequent pregnancy. Expectant parents will already be dealing with a flurry of emotions. They may get a positive test result more quickly than they were expecting and be surprised at how they are struck by both a sense of relief and happiness but also overwhelming guilt. They may immediately be worried about a loss of milk supply which is a common experience for many. They may have a strong sense of empathy for their child as they imagine how their world is going to change. They may be worried that their special relationship is going to change forever. They may even be focused on what is going to happen for the hours or days when they need to give birth and potentially be separated from them during labour. By continuing to breastfeed their toddler, they have already been up against it in terms of what most modern cultures find comfortable and acceptable. Now they are ticking the box for another misunderstood area of breastfeeding.

They may be told that their pregnancy is at risk. They may be told that they will be affecting the growth of their baby by 'taking away' their nutrition. They may be told they are 'using up' milk that the baby will need once they are born. It is all too easy for the myths to start dribbling out when the concept of breastfeeding the toddler in the first place was already poorly understood. Even when expressing the mildest level of concern, 'You're going to feel tired', the underlying assumption is one of 'Why bother?' Why would anyone bother to breastfeed when it no longer really matters? Parents are forced to justify themselves when they are at their most vulnerable. What does the research say about breastfeeding and pregnancy safety?

A study from 2012 looked at 320 women in Iran; some breastfed during pregnancy and some did not. It showed that:

> Results found no significant difference in full-term or non-full-term birth rates and mean newborn birth weight between the two groups. We further found no significant difference between full-term or non-full-term births and mean newborn birth weight for those who continued and discontinued breastfeeding during pregnancy in the overlap group. (Madarshahian and Hassanabadi 2012)

Breastfeeding during pregnancy didn't 'take nutrition away from the baby' and it did not cause prematurity.

In another study of 57 Californian women from 1993 (Moscone and Moore 1993), just under half continued to breastfeed through pregnancy and after the new baby arrived. The new babies were healthy and appropriately sized.

However, it is not all unequivocally positive. Another research study on 133 women in Peru found a link between breastfeeding through pregnancy and 125g on average less weight gain for the new baby in the first month (Marquis et al. 2002). Another study looked at 540 women in Egypt with sub-standard nutrition (Shaaban et al. 2015). This was not all positive news with increased risk of maternal anaemia and issues with infant growth. However, there was not an increase in miscarriage risk when women breastfed through pregnancy. It does appear that there might be an elevated risk to growth if parental nutritional levels and parental iron levels aren't sufficient.

A 2019 study did find a link between exclusive breastfeeding during pregnancy and miscarriage risk (Molitoris 2019). Exclusive breastfeeding here is meaning when breastfeeding is a nursling's only source of nutrition, that is, before the introduction of solid food. This study looked at nearly 11,000 pregnancies but did not distinguish between high- and low-risk pregnancies. It also found that there wasn't an increased risk once solid food had been introduced and the nurslings were presumably six months and older. This study was also based on historical interviews with parents from sometimes more than a decade ago rather than current medical observation.

Hilary Flower is the go-to person on the subject of breastfeeding during pregnancy. Her book *Adventures in Tandem Nursing* (2019) is considered the bible on this subject. Her focus was on bringing the facts to pregnant mothers and expectant families and she looked at this idea of triggering contractions or early labour in detail. She reminds us that we need oxytocin to trigger a milk ejection reflex (the letdown reflex) and this is also the hormone that can trigger uterine contractions. However, this doesn't mean that breastfeeding in pregnancy triggers risky contractions and there are several safeguards in place. We need hormone receptor sites to exist before hormones get acted on by the uterus, and they remain small in number until around 38 weeks of pregnancy. Even the hormone receptors that are in place cannot really do their job of causing contractions as there are oxytocin blockers in place like progesterone (made by the placenta) and proteins missing which would act as special agents to help the oxytocin do its job. Triple protection! So, oxytocin can carry on doing its breastfeeding job while baby remains protected in the uterus.

In her review of the 2019 Molitoris study, in an article written for La Leche League International with Gemma López, Hilary Flower says: 'Although it can be disconcerting to see the words breastfeeding, miscarriage, and risk all together like that, I believe there is no cause for alarm.' Flower and López suggest that there is 'perhaps' a reason to be concerned if a parent is exclusively breastfeeding: 'But this study leaves open the possibility that their risk may depend on their nutrition status and whether they have one of several "high risk" factors or pregnancy complications not controlled for in this study' (Flower and López 2019). More research is needed, but I think we can say science is on the side of those breastfeeding after six months and pregnant. This is certainly the view of the major health organizations of the world. Which makes sense when you think that throughout history women have been breastfeeding older babies and having sex and getting pregnant.

Dr Lesley Regan leads the Miscarriage Clinic at St Mary's Hospital in London, the largest referral unit in Europe, and is the author of *Miscarriage: What Every Woman Needs to Know* (Regan 2018a). She says: 'Once a pregnancy is clinically detectable, breastfeeding should pose no added risk of pregnancy loss. There isn't any data suggesting a link between breastfeeding and miscarriage, and I see no plausible reason for there to be a link' (Regan 2018b).

We can consider the history of pregnancy testing. Today, we might know we are pregnant days after conception. For generations, it was based on guesswork, someone examining your urine's appearance and something about rabbits (early 20th-century pregnancy tests involved injecting urine into a rabbit and observing a change in their ovaries). A lot of breastfeeding parents couldn't rely on whether they had missed a period as periods might only just be settling in or may not have even appeared yet. Some get pregnant without yet having a period. They 'catch the first egg'. Then they go and see their doctor and the doctor brings out the chart that predicts due date based on last menstrual period, 'Errr...2015?' Breastfeeding during pregnancy has been the norm for the vast majority of human history. It is still the norm in large parts of the world.

As one Italian-led review of the evidence stated:

> In Bangladesh in the late 1970s, more than 50% of the breastfeeding women who became pregnant continued to breastfeed beyond the sixth month of pregnancy. More recent data from Egypt indicate that 25% of women attending antenatal care conceive while breastfeeding. Among rural Guatemalans, 50% of pregnancies overlap with breastfeeding; moreover, 41% of women continue to breastfeed into the second trimester and 3% in the third trimester. In India, about 70% of mothers from poor urban and rural groups were still nursing when they became pregnant. (Monasta, Cetin and Davanzo 2014)

This review also concluded:

> The existence of a risk based on biological plausibility is not reason enough to dispense alarming advice and support compulsory weaning. It must be recognized that, as a whole, the potential negative consequences of breastfeeding during pregnancy on the health of the mother/embryo/fetus/nursed infant are not evidence based. On this basis, we can neither state that breastfeeding during pregnancy is always safe for the mother, the embryo, the fetus, and the toddler nor strongly support routine weaning to reduce risks that are not well documented at least in developed countries. Even in less developed countries, the risks related to overlapping breastfeeding and pregnancy seem to be associated more with the lack of sufficient nutrition of both the mother and the older child, with abrupt weaning, and with short intervals between births than with the overlapping itself. (Monasta *et al.* 2014)

There may be times when breastfeeding during pregnancy needs further discussion. The American Pregnancy Association states:

> While breastfeeding during pregnancy is generally considered safe, there are some cases where weaning may be advisable:
>
> - If you have a high-risk pregnancy or are at risk for preterm labor
> - If you are carrying twins
> - If you have been advised to avoid sex while pregnant
> - If you are having bleeding or uterine pain. (American Pregnancy Association 2017)

However, 'advisable' is still precautionary rather than in the face of robust scientific evidence, and each individual situation will need to be assessed separately with health professionals and families working together.

Of course, scientific evidence might suggest that breastfeeding during pregnancy is safe but that doesn't mean that everyone wishes to do it. As with all support we give to parents, we will need to ask open questions and help them reflect on what they want their journey to be. Some parents may be concerned about the experience of breastfeeding during pregnancy. Others may be more worried about the pressures of feeding two (or more) nurslings after pregnancy. The age of their current nursling may be a factor in their decision.

It is important that parents understand the implications if their child is under 12 months and still receiving breastmilk as a significant portion of their nutritional intake. It is highly likely that they will need to give an alternative source of milk. This will be different for every individual and it doesn't mean that breastfeeding has to end, but it is something that needs to be considered as the reduction in milk supply can be swift and unexpected for some. For parents who are passionate advocates of breastfeeding, it can be upsetting if their milk supply is hit hard during pregnancy, especially if their nursling is dependent nutritionally on their milk. In some cases, supplementing with an increase in solids and drinking water may be sufficient, but occasionally, families may be looking at formula for the first time. There may be families who prefer to access donor milk. Full fat cows' milk can only be given as a main drink after 12 months due to its micro-nutrient content and the protein load on young kidneys (Centers for Disease Control and Prevention 2018).

Most people who are breastfeeding when they are pregnant do notice a decrease in milk supply – often a very significant one. Most sources state that around 70% of parents will notice a supply drop (Flower 2019, p.92). This can start as early as the first few weeks after that positive pregnancy test. For some, it is an early indication of pregnancy. Whatever a parent does, their body will be re-setting in its lactation story and going back to making colostrum during pregnancy. It happens at different times and some people might go through a period of feeling like they have virtually nothing and their child is 'dry nursing' before colostrum then appears and quantities seem to increase again. In one study, around 18% described drying up completely for a stage of their pregnancy (Flower 2019, p.92).

Nurslings behave differently during the changes of pregnancy. Some self-wean as the quantities drop. Some self-wean when things seem to taste a bit different. Some care not a jot that changes are happening and would carry on breastfeeding whatever was coming out or if nothing was. Word of warning: colostrum has a laxative effect. That's one of the reasons it's so great for newborns as it helps them to pass meconium. If someone is potty training a toddler, they may need to be prepared!

Finding an online community can be powerful. If the community of those breastfeeding older children is small, it gets smaller again when we focus on those who are pregnant and breastfeeding older children (not least because the experience of pregnancy will only last a few months). Early posts may start with: 'I'm looking for reassurance that not everyone experiences a reduction in milk supply.' They may well find replies from the approximately 30% that don't (although they will have still re-set to colostrum during their pregnancy). Progesterone production increases in pregnancy as the breast tissue develops. The hormone performs multiple functions in pregnancy including managing the parent's immune response to enable acceptance of pregnancy, adjusting cervical mucus and optimizing the womb lining. Progesterone is often described as 'inhibiting lactation'. This is also the case post-partum if retained placental fragments were to remain, compromising the onset of copious milk production with their continued progesterone output. Hilary Flower suggests that progesterone may cause the milk storage areas to become more 'leaky' (Flower 2019, p.93). Certainly, the knowledge that both oestrogen and progesterone inhibit the stimulatory effects of prolactin is well established. Prolactin is made in pregnancy but there are processes that stop it doing its job. Progesterone interferes with prolactin binding to the receptors on the alveolar cells within the breast. There are also reservations around the use of hormonal contraception in early lactation.

The Infant Risk Center, one of the leading authorities on lactation and medication, states:

> We have no way to predict the outcome of breastfeeding once estrogen-containing birth control products are started. Some mothers may do fine and others can completely dry up. Therefore, if estrogen-containing contraception is chosen, it is advised that women use the lowest estrogen dosage appropriate and monitor their milk supply… Progesterone-only pills are preferred as they are less likely to decrease milk supply. Some women, however, are sensitive to even progesterone-only medications… (Infant Risk Center 2011)

It doesn't seem a leap to then expect progesterone and oestrogen in pregnancy to impact on supply.

The reduction in milk supply can be upsetting for some. It can come at a time when parents might already have mixed feelings about giving birth to another child. They may already be reflecting on a change in their nursling's life and a potential loss of their attention (even if another side of their brain understands what they will gain from a sibling). The loss of milk can feel doubly hard. Parents need to understand that there is little that can be done to increase supply in pregnancy once changes are observed. All the usual recommendations are no longer relevant: pumping, herbs, just feeding more frequently. Many herbs that we might consider when we want to increase production are not thought to be safe in pregnancy. Fenugreek, perhaps the most commonly used herbal galactagogue, is thought to be a uterine stimulant at medicinal doses (Bonyata 2018b). It is also true that many popular galactagogues report anecdotal success but the reasons for working are either poorly established or not understood. When there is a transformed hormonal profile, they may not work in the same way. Many galactagogues are thought to work by increasing oxytocin and prolactin. In pregnancy, the problem is not low levels of those hormones but higher levels of progesterone. The parents who are desperately searching for reassurance that their supply won't decrease would best be served by a realistic message that it is very likely that it will, and that they and their nursling will be OK.

It's important to remember though (and this is engraved on the heart of many of us in breastfeeding support) that BREASTFEEDING IS NOT JUST ABOUT MILK and this is a message we can emphasize when supporting pregnant parents. If nutrition and milk intake is the concern, parents may want to consider using a supplementary feeding system at the breast, so baby can remain attached and get other milk through a lightweight tube. Many nurslings will continue even when their nutritional needs are not being met at the breast. Even when 'dry nursing' (apparently no milk is being transferred), a nursling will happily remain attached and the breast very much continues to be home, providing comfort and reassurance and relaxation.

Other than supply reduction, there are some other symptoms noted by many, but not all, parents. Sore nipples can be an issue and it appears this is due to a hormonal sensitivity, similar to what some experience at certain points in their menstrual cycle. There may also be breast sensitivity. Aversion may develop as a result of hyperemesis gravidarum (HG) (severe and persistent nausea during pregnancy).

> Breastfeeding with HG was very hard, especially because I began to experience breastfeeding aversion too, but it felt so important to keep going, in part so my older daughter didn't feel like it was the baby's fault or the illness's fault that she didn't get her milky. I had to push through and I'm glad I did. I went on sick leave from work and spent most of my time in bed or on the sofa. Fi took charge of all the childcare and household tasks, while also holding down her own job. Without her, I wouldn't have made it through this second pregnancy.
>
> What helped me during HG, besides my wife Fi's care, was:
>
> - Viewing breastfeeding as a chance to rest (since you can sit or lie down), which is very important when ill with HG.
> - Since smells bothered me, we avoided scented soaps/shampoos/lotions generally and, if necessary, Esther would wash up before coming for a feed.
> - Reading to Esther while breastfeeding. This worked well because sometimes I needed distraction from my nausea or breastfeeding aversion. It also helped me feel like I was still a mother, even though I couldn't parent in the ways I usually did.
> - Sometimes, when I was very nauseated or suffering from aversion or both, I had to limit breastfeeding either to the length of a particular song or book, or to count down the time we would spend feeding, so I still got the closeness with my child but knew that I wouldn't be suffering uncomfortably for too long.
> - I kept reminding myself that Esther might be angry or upset about my pregnancy or my illness, and that breastfeeding was a

> wonderful way of keeping our connection going and to help her deal with her big feelings.
>
> ~ (BJ Woodstein)

Once baby is here, a family enters a new phase of tandem feeding. The term 'tandem feeding' simply means 'feeding two' and it can be used to refer to someone who is pregnant who is providing nutrition to both an internal and external child. Triandem feeding refers to feeding three children at the same time. This might include a family with one set of twins or a newborn, toddler and pre-schooler. You can also find families describing their quadandem journey online.

How does breastfeeding work when there is a newborn and a toddler? While breastfeeding during pregnancy doesn't 'use up' colostrum, it's sensible to let the newborn do their thing first before the older nursling gets a turn. Colostrum volumes are smaller and a newborn should have first access before an older child can provide additional stimulation to a newly developing milk supply. Once colostrum transitions to mature milk, decisions can be based on how the newborn's nappies and weight gain are getting on. Sometimes there is talk of restricting a baby to one breast and a toddler to another. Most lactation consultants agree that is not sensible. Ideally, we would want the newborn to have the option of both breasts and continue to have the option of both fully lactating as their breastfeeding experience continues. Restricting a toddler to one side may mean that 'their' breast reduces in volume, turns to produce 'weaning milk' (which is different in composition) and eventually dries. All this while the newborn is continuing its breastfeeding journey. Swapping sides regularly also means the newborn has symmetrical visual stimulation (rather than having one eye effectively blinkered for a significant portion of the day). It also means that the newborn has options should one breast develop mastitis or become painful or damaged. Toddlers feeding after newborns are very effective at helping a milk supply to develop, and tipping into over-supply is more of a worry than running out of milk. A toddler is also fabulous at relieving engorgement in the early days post-partum and this is one of the advantages of tandem feeding.

Does the toddler feel jealous of the baby having 'their milk'? I have yet to meet a parent who feels that's been a significant problem. In fact, many feel that it can help in the arrival of a new member of the family. Everyone benefits from the regular doses of oxytocin – a hormone which is known to aid relationship building and bonding. Toddlers are likely to need some extra support, but breastfeeding is still there for them – the thing that has always provided comfort and reassurance. And good news! It's changing back to regular milk and there's lots more of it! What might not be sensible is weaning a toddler in the last few weeks of pregnancy, so if a parent feels tandem breastfeeding really isn't for them, it might be wiser to wean sooner rather than just prior to baby arriving. Trying to wean an older nursling when there is also a young baby feeding is likely to be challenging, not least because the parent is going to be sensitized to the possibility the older child may feel rejected. However, nothing is impossible, and if feeding an older child alongside a newborn feels unmanageable, the parent can be supported to make changes. An older child can appreciate that their needs are different and they are able to eat an exciting wider range of foods. What may help is a visual representation of all the months (or weeks) they have breastfed throughout their life compared to the weeks their sibling has fed. You might represent each week with a coloured block. A much older child might even be interested in considering gallons or litres. They may feel as though they are missing out but really they have had an impressive stint. They may be satisfied with small amounts of milk in a cup, that feeding is still 'cuddle time' or a very short feed for only a few seconds in a transitional phase. They may protest at the thought of milk ending and, as with any aspect of weaning, these emotions can be explored and validated rather than avoided. I once heard someone describe the arrival of a new sibling as being like your spouse announcing that they were going to bring in a third member of the marriage against your will and you WERE going to love them and accept them. We often hear parents say, 'But I don't want them to be jealous of the baby.' What may be more helpful is to acknowledge that jealousy may be natural; we can't control those emotions but we can show we are there for them in different ways. If breastfeeding wasn't in the picture, it is likely there would be another focus for resentment and exploring boundaries. If a parent is struggling to breastfeed an older child and doing so through gritted teeth, it is unlikely that that helps to create a positive environment for the new dynamics of a family. It is possible for them to put limits in place as well as fully wean if they wish to.

It sometimes happens that an older child who hasn't breastfed for a while asks to do so again when a new baby is on the scene. That might be because they weren't a fan of the colostrum or there might be some other things going on in their head. Are they testing whether they still get to be your baby? Are they just curious? Some resume breastfeeding at this point. Some are happy to have a taste of expressed milk in a cup. Some ask and run away giggling and don't mention it again. There's no right or wrong answer on how to deal with this, but ideally, we're looking for ways to minimize rejection, and so any refusal should be given as gently as possible.

> My fertility returned very quickly after Nicola was born and I became pregnant quite soon after. I have breastfed through my pregnancy. I felt quite tired so I used to have a rest when she was having her nap. I was planning to tandem feed, but she self-weaned at about 20 months old when I was approaching eight months of my pregnancy. At the time it felt like a bit of a relief but once Sasha was born I was sad that I couldn't feed them both. Nicola tried to come onto the breast but she just didn't know how to suck any more. So I squirted some milk into her mouth a few times. I never refused her when she tried to come over and have a cuddle with me and baby. She was only 22 months. Soon she started bringing her dolls and breastfeeding them next to me while I breastfed Sasha. Just precious.
>
> ~ *(Miriam Feen)*

When it comes to talking about breastfeeding in pregnancy and risk, there may be another way to look at the situation. The American Academy of Family Physicians states:

> Breastfeeding during a subsequent pregnancy is not unusual. If the pregnancy is normal and the mother is healthy, breastfeeding during pregnancy is the woman's personal decision. If the child is younger than two years, the child is at increased risk of illness if weaned.
>
> Breastfeeding the nursing child during pregnancy and after delivery of the next child (tandem nursing) may help provide a smooth transition psychologically for the older child. (American Academy of Family Physicians 2014)

So, as is often the case in conversations around infant feeding, we may need to reverse our language. Perhaps we should be thinking in terms of the risk of ending breastfeeding earlier than was planned or the potential risk in *not* continuing to breastfeed. That's not to say that parental choice isn't always top of the agenda, but a child whose parent falls pregnant at eight months will likely have a minimum of double the breastfeeding duration if they are enabled to tandem feed and continue to feed during pregnancy. Breastfeeding continues to offer 'significant nutritional and immunological benefits' and 'better social adjustment' (American Academy of Family Physicians 2014).

Of course, all this discussion means a parent has got pregnant. Trying to conceive while pregnant, or trying to avoid conceiving when pregnant, takes up a lot of thinking too.

If a parent is exclusively breastfeeding and responsively breastfeeding (not trying to feed on a schedule but seeing breastfeeding as a multifaceted comfort and sleep tool), has not seen a return of their menstrual cycle and baby is under six months old, breastfeeding is considered a reliable contraceptive method. As mentioned earlier, this is known as the lactational amenorrhoea method. However, as this book discusses breastfeeding beyond six months, this method is no longer considered reliable. The message that breastfeeding initially prevents conception may give the misleading impression that continued breastfeeding continues that prevention but parents need to be supported to consider other methods. This may include natural family planning methods, sometimes known as fertility awareness methods. This is best done with professional support as some of the markers can be more challenging to assess when breastfeeding (e.g. taking a morning temperature when a night's sleep may have been more disrupted, or assessing ovulation signs). Barrier methods are also popular. Methods using hormones may be more problematic and, as mentioned earlier, some parents do notice a reduction in their milk supply. As the American Academy of Family Physicians states:

> many anecdotal reports link hormonal contraceptives to a decrease in milk supply, and a Cochrane review found that the data are inconsistent and limited. In particular, many of the studies do not consider exclusivity of breastfeeding. (American Academy of Family Physicians 2014)

This may even be the case for progestin (progesterone)-only methods, despite the fact they are usually considered safer. However, as we are talking about those breastfeeding beyond six months, we are likely to be dealing with parents who have a more established milk supply and are at less risk. Concerns may remain for parents with a history of breast or chest surgery or where there have been concerns around weight gain in the past.

For those who want to conceive, an end to breastfeeding may not be necessary. When the menstrual cycle does return (on average at around 14 months) (Bonyata 2018c), it may not be predictable and may fluctuate according to nursing patterns. It may be triggered by a baby or toddler sleeping for a longer period, but the pattern may change again as nursing patterns shift.

It may be that a period has returned but without full fertility. This may be because ovulation is not occurring or there is a short luteal phase (the gap between ovulation and the menstrual bleed). If there is a short luteal phase, this may mean there isn't sufficient time for implantation to be fully established after fertilization. Parents who wish to conceive, but don't wish to give up breastfeeding entirely, may look at reducing breastfeeding frequency or night-weaning initially. It does appear that a more abrupt change can kick-start a return to fertility, rather than a gradual shift, but that may not always sit comfortably alongside gentle parenting methods. There is a myth that the effectiveness of pregnancy tests is impacted by breastfeeding, but the hormone being detected, human chorionic gonadotropin, is unaffected by breastfeeding. If you are supporting someone who is trying to conceive while breastfeeding, an important message is that everyone is different. There is no universal amount of breastfeeding that means full fertility returns, nor length of time post-partum. They will need to be supported to learn more about the signs of ovulation and to make their own decisions about their breastfeeding journey.

Some parents will have conceived initially with an assisted conception and be looking to return to the clinic for a sibling, or they may be thinking about IVF for a subsequent pregnancy. There is a perception that this method of conception will require a complete end to breastfeeding, but this isn't a perception supported by scientific evidence.

Ali Thomas started the Facebook group 'Breastfeeding mums undergoing fertility treatment/IVF' around six years ago. She spends around 20 to 30 hours a week volunteering on the group, alongside her small team of admin volunteers, as well as working full-time as an environmental health officer in Nottingham, England.

> I started the group for myself as I had had IVF to conceive my daughter. As we started to think about using one of our frozen embryos, I didn't want to stop breastfeeding. I was already a mother supporter/peer supporter for the Association of Breastfeeding Mothers and I

knew my stuff and how much I wanted to continue to feed until natural term, so I started to do some research. What I found out is that there was literally nothing. I found one podcast from an Australian breastfeeding counsellor. That was it. That was the only thing available on the entire internet. I decided if there wasn't any support out there, I would start it.

The group started with three members and now we have 4000 from all over the world. We have a strict joining process for our support group with a screening process. There is a public-facing website and Facebook page but they signpost to the private group for support. Other resources signpost to the group like the Drugs in Breastmilk service factsheet written by Wendy Jones MBE, the specialist pharmacist with the Breastfeeding Network. She does sit within the group to occasionally answer queries about medication and offer next level support. We're also signposted to by the National Breastfeeding Helpline and organizations like La Leche League.

At the start it was heart-breaking because all I ever came across was women who had already weaned and then suddenly realized they didn't have to. That is really the hardest part – people finding us too late.

Families are often told by staff in fertility clinics that they have to wean. The majority attitude is that you should stop breastfeeding for fertility treatment. Breastfeeding is seen as something that's not really necessary. These mums will usually have older children and why would you be thinking about continuing to breastfeed? You don't need to. Every clinic seems to have a different reason and we do collate that data and people share their experiences on the group. It's so random. Some clinics say you have to have weaned for four weeks before starting treatment. Some say three months. Some say six months. Some say it's because the medications are dangerous. Some say it's because you'll have a higher risk of miscarriage. Some say it's because your prolactin levels will be too high which will impact on the medication, although if they test they are likely to find someone breastfeeding an older child has normal prolactin levels. There is no one reason. There is no national or international guidance on breastfeeding alongside fertility treatment, although clinic groups may develop their own breastfeeding stance. The Human Fertilisation and Embryology Authority (HFEA) governs clinics in the UK but doesn't have a position on breastfeeding.

Often someone will have treatment at a clinic and not disclose they are breastfeeding. That's what I did personally. I was told I had to wean and come back after three months of no breastfeeding. I contacted the clinic again three months later and they never asked. Often if someone has a two- or three-year-old, they are just not asked. It is a quandary for some people. Even if they have done their research, they don't like the idea of not telling the truth. We do empower people to challenge their clinic in the group if that's what they want to do. Some will do that successfully. They will take information from respected sources like LactMed, e-lactancia, Infantrisk.org. It can also be useful to signpost the clinics that do allow continued breastfeeding. We have breastfeeding-friendly clinics, breastfeeding-tolerant clinics and anti-breastfeeding clinics. Australia seems to do better with breastfeeding acceptance. UK is behind and hardly anywhere in the USA is breastfeeding-friendly. Some of our members will travel abroad for treatment. Costs may be lower with shorter waiting lists. They may find a more breastfeeding-friendly culture elsewhere, for example UK families may travel to other European countries like Poland, the Czech Republic and Portugal. In the last five years, I have seen an increase in the number of supportive clinics. There is a small change in the tide.

Clinics assume breastfeeding will impact on success rate without having done any research. As profit-driven businesses, they are looking for rates of success that improve footfall, so a blanket ban feels less risky. It's easy to cut any perceived risk if you don't understand the value of breastfeeding, but there is no evidence that breastfeeding does affect IVF success. There has been no research but we do know we see a lot of successes in the group.

In the group, some people are celebrating successes and births and others are experiencing losses. In some IVF groups, birth posts aren't allowed without trigger warnings, but we are set up to advertise our success, that is, 'You can conceive with IVF while breastfeeding', so people tend to have more tolerance. However, we do manage our group carefully and have specific areas for specific topics.

It does come up a lot that parents are told they miscarried because they are breastfeeding, again with no evidence to back that up and on an untested embryo. There is one small study that links breastfeeding and a small increase in miscarriage but that is when conception happens in the first six months post-partum and with high-risk pregnancies. This isn't relevant to our group as someone is rarely resuming IVF after less than six months.

Sometimes we need to re-set expectations around breastfeeding and natural fertility. It's common for periods to not have returned at nine months but clinics won't always understand that.

If you have gone to such lengths to conceive, you are likely to be hit hard by miscarriage, not to say that it's easy for anyone. But there is no automatic 'trying again' when it costs such lengths. You might need £8000 or more to try again. A transfer of a frozen embryo from a previous round will still be several thousand pounds.

Other options include medications to induce ovulation: clomid, letrozole and metformin. Using these drugs can be harder when you are breastfeeding than a regular IVF round. Letrozole is contraindicated when breastfeeding. Clomid is complicated. It used to be that if letrozole was contraindicated, people moved to clomid, but then some sources changed to say it may not be compatible with breastfeeding. None of these drugs are licensed for breastfeeding, so you are always looking at different sources to reach a decision. Some people will contact Rodney White in Australia for further information. Others go to the Infant Risk forum or UKDILAS (UK Drugs in Lactation Advisory Service). They will need individual information based on their personal situation.

Partners will vary in their level of support. Some will also automatically push for weaning to happen like a fertility clinic. Others will be more understanding of the value of the breastfeeding relationship. Often the group is just an ear. These are people who not only have the complications of the breastfeeding journey but also the fertility journey which is hard emotionally and physically. There is a lot going on. Then on top of your stress of the journey, you are taking these hormonal medications. They further impact on your emotions. A lot of the work in the group is about passing a virtual hanky and listening to someone cry online. The website is useful to signpost other people to but the group is very private and just for people going through the journey themselves. We don't have observers or health professional members as that feels a little voyeuristic.

Breastfeeding often matters more to people going through a fertility journey. The conception has been totally medicalized. Everything is done according to a clock and under the control of others. Breastfeeding becomes so important as you want to take something back for yourself, something not measured and controlled. IVF can mean you lose faith in your body, so a lot of these people are broken emotionally because they feel like their bodies are broken, but breastfeeding can give them their faith in their body back again. You can do everything to nurture a baby; just because you couldn't make the baby on your own, it doesn't mean you can't do everything else.

In this group, I don't often meet people who want to wean. They all really, really care about breastfeeding. They all really want to keep going. They see the benefit of feeding to natural term. In considering fertility treatment, they can feel a tear when asked to stop breastfeeding. Do they want to stop just for the chance of another child? If an IVF cycle has only a 30% success rate, how guilty will you feel afterwards if you've stopped and your treatment has been unsuccessful? A lot of people take comfort from continuing breastfeeding when their treatment hasn't worked. They can cuddle up with their two-year-old and think, 'At least I didn't stop.' That is commonly a way people will comfort themselves after a failed cycle. It's certainly how I felt after a failed cycle and a miscarriage. I thought, 'Thank goodness I didn't force my daughter to stop breastfeeding.'

Fertility medications are hormonal, and even if they aren't unsafe with breastfeeding, they might lead to a reduction in milk supply. We need to communicate to people to be cautious if they are breastfeeding a baby under 12 months who may rely on breastfeeding for nutrition. It's true of pregnancy too – milk supply can reduce.

I wish health professionals understood there is a value in breastfeeding and they shouldn't just dismiss it. They should do their research. The stark difference between the clinics that 'allow' breastfeeding and the ones that don't is that the ones that allow it have done their research and looked into the medication. It is such a simple thing to do. They also need to remember people are paying for this service, thousands of pounds, and it is their choice. It's my body, my choice and I'm giving you my hard-earned money. I want to do what I want to do. They are disempowering us at a time when we already feel massively disempowered. Fertility treatment is already disempowering. It can already make you feel bad about yourself and they are adding to the emotional load. A little bit of research will tell them how valuable it is and how possible it is. If I can do the research with no medical training, I think they can look into it, and support families, too.

~ *(Ali Thomas)*

Pregnancy can sometimes bring the end of breastfeeding. Not every nursling wishes to dry nurse or continue with the transition to colostrum. Not every parent wishes to continue through aversion and nipple sensitivity. Whatever triggers the end of breastfeeding, even when a new baby and a new breastfeeding experience is imminent, their emotional reaction may take a parent by surprise. This can be a time when parents are already feeling finely tuned to how their child's life is going to change and the end of their babyhood.

> I weaned J shortly after her third birthday when I was about 15 weeks pregnant with O. I have mixed feelings about this. I weaned her because pregnancy gave me horrible nipple pain and vasospasm. She was down to just a feed at bedtime and it was very short when we stopped – perhaps 30 seconds or so. My milk had pretty much gone by then anyway. I was relieved in many ways to stop as I found it so painful at the end, but I also felt really sad that it had ended at my direction rather than hers. I had really wanted the weaning to be led by her. We swapped a bedtime feed for a bedtime story and cuddle and it wasn't traumatic for her. But she very clearly wasn't ready to wean as she continued to occasionally ask for milk for months afterwards, especially if tired or upset. She also still has a dummy overnight so evidently she still has a need to suck. Overall I feel immensely proud of my breastfeeding experience with her, but the end is definitely tinged with sadness.
>
> ~ *(Naomi Dow)*

For parents

The poem on the next page by Dr Victoria Thomas captures some of the emotions parents often have when they are pregnant and still nursing:

Cuckoo

You curl around the curve of my belly,
taut as a bow drawn to fire the arrow
that will be your sister.
Eight months pregnant,
Nothing is comfortable for me now.
Even breathing feels laborious.
But you are here to find the comfort in my body
as natural as breathing to you.
One child within, one child outside,
Hug through my flesh.
Deep breath.
You lift your face and squeak indignantly
'There's not much milk.' My heart stutters.
I don't want you to resent her before she's even here.
Our longed-for cuckoo in your comfy nest.
I take your hand.
'The baby will bring more milk when she's born.'
'She will?' Your face lights up. You glow.
You bend your head and kiss the bump
'Oh thank you baby.'
They bring their own love, I think
We'll be OK, I know.

Chapter 10

Ending Breastfeeding

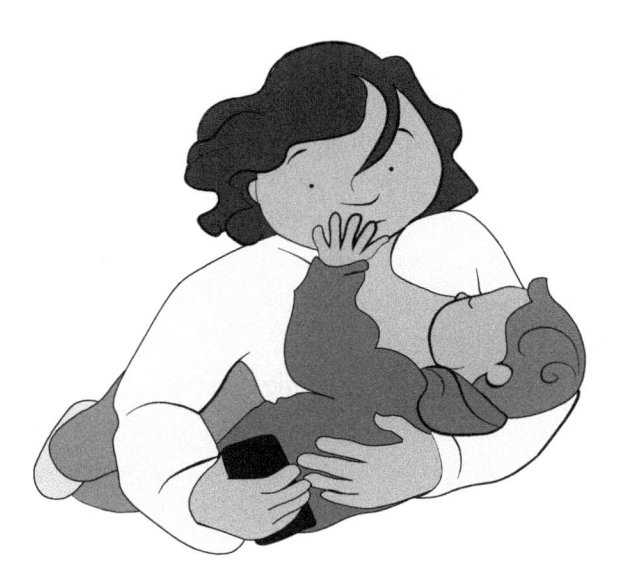

There are as many different ways to end breastfeeding as there are nursing families. It can be easy to make an assumption that those who continue to breastfeed beyond 12 months will inevitably end up practising child-led weaning and avoid using parent-led weaning methods, but these sort of assumptions can leave parents feeling unsupported and isolated.

As we know, continuing to breastfeed beyond the second and third years can be socially isolating and many parents come to rely on social media groups, but sometimes there the support is focused on normalizing continuing. A focus on weaning/ending breastfeeding is not always a comfortable area for discussion. It can be difficult to support an individual parent to wean at 14 months, for example, alongside the narrative that a 14-month-old is genuinely in their early days of breastfeeding, and weaning between three and seven years is the norm. A parent who wishes to wean before 18 months may feel they have a limited range of support on offer. This is not to say that members of social media communities lack empathy or are full of individuals who are purely self-serving, but that it is a very challenging balance to get right in what is essentially a community all having mutual conversations spoken out loud within the earshot of the thousands of members.

Weaning older children can be messy. If it is parent-initiated, it can mean a tension between a parent's self-protection and the wishes of their child. If a parent has issues with anxiety, this can feel like a period of uncertainty and unpredictability. Routines will be changing and adaptation is needed. A parent may be concerned about a shift in their identity. They may feel as though they are saying goodbye to a part of themselves and a community they have come to value. When social media may mean that daily conversation revolves around their identity as a breastfeeding parent, the next stage can feel hard to visualize. For autistic nurslings, the end of breastfeeding is likely to bring more challenges and the family will need greater support. They may, for example, struggle more with a change to routine and a loss of a familiar strategy that helps with emotional regulation. There are few parenting decisions where a parent can feel as guilty putting their own needs first. They may intellectually appreciate that their child benefits from a peaceful and happy end to the breastfeeding relationship for both parent and child, but it doesn't feel any easier when the nursling is crying at 2 am and pleading for the breast.

There are some families who may wish for an end to breastfeeding but decide to continue, even when they find the situation challenging and stressful. Dr Sally Dowling:

> A lot of people I spoke to said that they carried on because of the child and that it was the child's will. They couldn't imagine stopping because they couldn't imagine how they could have that kind of conflict with the child. They were doing it because the child wanted it and needed it but they were exhausted and stressed. I was quite surprised by how many described a negative experience. Personally, I also found it really difficult. I had my last two children in my forties – I last breastfed when I was 47! – and I was tired and often unwell and my youngest didn't sleep for many years. I think she was 11 when she slept through. When I look back on that time, it was really hard but it was also one of the most amazing things I've done, and I think you can have those two feelings co-existing. I couldn't have done it without the support of my partner, who absolutely got it, and in the early months, without LLL (La Leche League).
>
> ~ *(Dr Sally Dowling)*

As supporters of breastfeeding families, we need to provide a space for conversations that allow parents to express their frustration and distress but don't assume that they are simply hoping for a validation to be able to start the weaning process. There is not a single parent who is feeding an older child who does not appreciate that the concept of parent-led weaning exists in the world. Certainly, there may be some conversations where a parent is edging towards making a decision to wean and is looking for a chance to explore those feelings. However, we must be careful to ensure we don't rush to assumptions where we feel a conversation may be heading that way. There are also a lot of parents who are struggling but do not intend to wean and need us to appreciate that choice and the complexity around it. If it is not always easy for parents to find a space where they can talk about parent-led weaning, it can be even harder to find a space to talk about the desire not to wean in the face of a struggle that most would consider unmanageable. It is possible for a parent to be miserable, resentful, exhausted and in pain and still not want to wean and for them to need someone to understand that is their right. What other support can we offer?

When weaning is a hope, professionals can facilitate the pros and cons conversation and discuss what feels challenging and what they hope weaning may bring. This can be important as sometimes there may be false assumptions that weaning ALWAYS means a toddler sleeping through the night or an easier bedtime or is required for a return to fertility. These are conversations where we must exercise our top skills in empathy and avoid projection. That is as much true for the breastfeeding counsellor who breastfed for five years as it is for the professional who stopped at three months. Because parent-led weaning of older children is rarely discussed in detail, there may not be realistic expectations of the likely timeframe and there may also be an assumption that the ultimate aim is to try and avoid the nursling being upset. In truth, one of the first conversations needed may be around the fact that their nursling has the right to mourn the end of the breastfeeding relationship as much as parents have the right to their own body autonomy and the ability to choose to bring breastfeeding to a close. Certainly, there are times when we can look for distraction and attempt to avoid a sense of rejection. It's always the ideal to naturally avoid tears and upset, but the idea that successful weaning means a toddler peacefully acquiescing, and anything less than this is cruelty, is unhelpful. If a nursling is expressing anger and frustration, these can be opportunities for validation and understanding, rather than a scrabbled desperate time to switch off those emotions. Helping a child to come to terms with the loss of breastfeeding with discussion and open dialogue is a powerful parenting opportunity. Supporting a child through loss gives a valuable opportunity to explore their resilience. Far from this all being a quest to find an end to breastfeeding with the least emotional reaction possible, it is about looking for the emotions and supporting through them. We want little people to feel they can express anger and sadness at the loss of breastfeeding. We even want the big people to be able to say that they feel sad too. There is an option for both the parent and the nursling to have their own rites of passage ceremony where they say goodbye to nursing and talk about what was special, share memories and record them for posterity. It can be helpful when speaking to an older nursling to highlight that this is a change for both of you. Rather than the child being the only one experiencing loss, both parent and child are entering a new phase. Replacing the phrase 'You don't have milkies any more' with 'We don't have milkies any more' or 'Mummy and Alfie don't have milkies any more' immediately changes the dynamic. Talking is important. Even young children respond well to preparation, and a reminder that tonight the pattern of bedtime will be different can be scattered throughout a day and talked about in different moments. A nursling is more likely to feel ownership if change is not sprung on them unexpectedly. Each parent will have a sense of how best to approach the transition.

We sometimes hear talk of weaning parties: balloons and cakes that look like breasts. That may be a positive celebration for an older child ending their breastfeeding experience, but are parties 'allowed' to contain some sadness? We want space for the entire range of emotions.

A weaning celebration doesn't have to be a party but an opportunity for reflection and to mark the significance of the event:

> A few weeks ago, I stopped breastfeeding my youngest child. She will be five years old in a couple of weeks. We came to the decision together and it felt like the right time for both of us. To mark the occasion, I asked her what she would like to do for our Weaning Celebration. She requested, 'A new park and ice cream!' So today we went out for a gorgeous afternoon together and it was [the] most perfect day. We came across a secluded orchard with a little table under a beautiful tree of blossom which we sat at together. I read a card I had written to her about what our breastfeeding journey has meant to me and how our relationship is changing now but how our bond will always be there. And then I surprised her with her weaning

> gift – a locket with our photos inside. She gifted me back some fallen blossom in the box. We had our ice cream. We visited a small farm where very fittingly we saw a lot of lovely breastfeeding amongst calves and piglets (with their respective mothers!). And we wandered and explored and just celebrated being together.
>
> ~ *(Laura)*

Even if we are passionate supporters of breastfeeding for several years, being a breastfeeding advocate means supporting a parent to end breastfeeding whenever they wish to. If this doesn't happen, and breastfeeding beyond 12 months is seen as silently signing a contract to breastfeeding for several more years, breastfeeding even younger babies may be at risk. It will be attractive to end breastfeeding at eight months if there is apparently no method and support network if you wish to end breastfeeding at 13 months. I have been told by the editorial team of an attachment parenting magazine that they never print articles about parent-led weaning and few Instagram influencers breastfeeding beyond two years will be openly sharing their parent-led weaning experiences. Recently, a mother posted on Facebook to show the photo of her first and last feed (where she was in tears). Rather than being met with universal support, there were several posters who scolded her for practising parent-led weaning and congratulated themselves for not doing so. Even if we wish child-led weaning for every nursling in the bottom of our hearts, we must acknowledge this isn't right for every parent: those experiencing aversion, survivors of sexual assault, those with medical issues, those who simply wish to stop. We need to normalize breastfeeding ending at any age if we want to normalize breastfeeding at any age.

Family members may also feel if a parent has chosen to continue, they have 'made their own bed' and not feel they can offer much practical support. Too often, parents who continue feeding say that they have stopped reaching out for help. It feels as though they have lost permission to be able to explain that they are struggling or that they have hard days or that they are feeling tired. If someone has had a year or more of not reaching out, when weaning time does come around, they may not feel in the mood to ask for help. If the response is going to be 'Finally!' rather than 'Well done for feeding as long as you have. You must be really proud. How can I help?', a parent may wish to keep their decision to themselves.

Regular breastfeeding peer support may not have sufficient experience in ending breastfeeding with toddlers and older children. We need to speak up if this is an area where we can offer support. It is good practice if you are a peer supporter who did not breastfeed for an extended period of time to have a resources bank that includes those who breastfed through pregnancy, fed into toddlerhood and beyond and understand both parent-led and more child-led weaning. If you are a health professional, you may be more accustomed to signposting to peer support. Some parents have not made it publicly known that they are still breastfeeding, so looking for support during the weaning stage may mean going public when they least feel able. It may also be the case the breastfeeding drop-ins centre around young babies. There are practical challenges with bringing a mobile older nursling into that environment and also sometimes psychological ones.

Whether weaning is child-led or parent-led is not a distinction we need to spend a lot of time analysing. It may be unrealistic to imagine that 'pure' child-led weaning is ever technically possible for most of us. Few families operate in circumstances where a child isn't offered a separate sleeping space at some point, other food or drink or there is no return to work or other types of separation (including caring for younger siblings). The weaning experience begins the moment other nutrition is around, which is why the term 'weaning' has confusingly come to mean both the introduction of solid food and the end of breastfeeding. The end of breastfeeding may take many, many years but the process starts for most at around six months. Is this child-led technically? Does it matter? Even the parents who feel passionately committed to child-led weaning may sometimes nudge a feed to end, request a delay or offer an alternative activity and this is natural and normal.

If a parent has been told that they need to end breastfeeding in order to have medical treatment or to take medications, this is something that will need careful research. As most of us who support breastfeeding families are all too familiar with, drug manufacturers may not always undergo trials on breastfeeding parents, but reliable evidence may exist which confirms that medications can be compatible with breastfeeding, even when the manufacturer's literature may not suggest this. If a drug is deemed to be unsafe, an alternative can often be found. For parents with a history of mental health issues, it is particularly important that they are supported to breastfeed for as long as they wish. There is sometimes a view that when a parent is under pressure or struggling in other ways, the ending of breastfeeding will bring some relief, but the loss of regular doses of oxytocin may have a negative impact. Parents can also be surprised at the sense of loss that can come with the end of breastfeeding, even when it is something they had full control over. The hormonal shifts will affect some more than others. It can also bring up emotions about the entire breastfeeding journey and it's important that parents are supported and have an opportunity to speak to someone who understands and has time to listen. 'Weaning blues' is a relatively common experience:

> I found the process of stopping breastfeeding quite difficult this time around. I remember feeling some sadness when my son stopped feeding just after his first birthday, but somehow it was compounded this time. I believe there were probably a few factors that impacted this. Firstly, I think that because she was exclusively breastfed (my son was 90% breastfeeding but had a bottle each night), I had the impression that she would continue longer. At about nine months she was still feeding regularly both day and night and I couldn't see that stopping. So there was a grief process of managing my own expectations there for sure. Secondly, she was born into a year when everybody stayed home, all the time. She had only ever known me, my husband and son, and lately one set of grandparents. Her attachment to me is

strong, she spent the first five months of her life also permanently attached to me, either feeding or in a sling and has never experienced any of the hallmarks of a first year, no relatives, playgroups or days out. I am all she knows! Lastly, she is most likely to be our last baby, and so the thought of never feeding again seems more final in a way.

I also had a small feeling of no longer being 'in the club'. I can no longer partake in those conversations where mums complain about their baby 'feeding all the time'...etc., etc. Although we moan, there's an underlying sense of pride that you are still breastfeeding, despite it being hard! I reached out to friends who have also had babies this year and we had several WhatsApp chats around the subject. I also received a beautiful hand-drawn card from a friend which read 'breastfeeding, loved, completed' – I have to say, this did make me weep a little!

~ *(Laura, a UK midwife whose breastfeeding journey ended when her daughter was 11 months)*

I was pregnant and/or breastfeeding for eight consecutive years, and though weaning was gradual and child-led (with some compassionate nursing limits sprinkled in at the appropriate times), I was not prepared for the neuroendocrine hurricane that would ravage my mental health once our journey was complete. I'd experienced baby blues and had my fair share of anxiety during parenthood, but because my 'baby' was weaning at four and a half years, I thought I was 'out of the woods' and wouldn't experience any depressive episodes this late in the game. Because I'd been working with families in a professional helping context for almost as long as my first child had been alive, I knew to expect some sadness, guilt and feelings of ambiguity about the changing relationship and I expected to grieve the transition, but I did not expect the plummeting lows and mood fluctuations that would leave me crumpled crying in the corner of the laundry room contemplating whether my kids would be better off without me. And while I was aware that the shifts in mood were hormonally mediated, I don't have a history of depression, I couldn't change my feelings (even with the usual mindfulness and meditation strategies) and I had neither any idea how long to expect the storm to last nor the internal compass to navigate my way through.

About four weeks after my son stopped nursing daily, the depressive symptoms began to snowball and for about four weeks I was unrecognizable, even to myself. My husband literally picked me up from the corner of the laundry room (more than once), dusted me off, and helped me put one foot in front of the other until things began to make a little more sense.

Weaning emotions are more than feelings. What's happening is a complex biological process that's as much hormonal and psychological as it is social and physical. The relaxation caused by prolactin and the cosy connection associated with oxytocin decrease as oestrogen and progesterone rise, which can affect the production and transport of neurotransmitters in regions of the brain related to emotion.

Ultimately, the things that helped me most were talk therapy; research, understanding and targeted use of neurotransmitter supplements; anxiolytic herbs, exercise, rest and focus on nutrition. I'm not sure what makes certain genotypes more susceptible/vulnerable to the mental and emotional 'hi-jacking' that occurs with hormonal fluctuations or how to prevent bouts of depression and the feelings of rage, anxiety, hopelessness and helplessness that some of us embody during even gradual weaning, but I hope that as the science in our field continues to advance we will have a better understanding of how to help on both neuro-chemical and interpersonal levels in a way that validates our experiences, embraces our vulnerabilities, holds space during the darkness and utilizes a functional approach to help balance and restore so that we can be our best selves for us and for our children.

~ *(Amy, who stopped breastfeeding when her son was four and a half years)*

Weaning blues are not a well-researched area but a few minutes in a breastfeeding support group online will make it clear they are a widely recognized experience. As Laura mentions, there can be a sense that a part of the parent's identity has been lost, especially if this was a last baby. Parents may need to develop new skills, whether that is helping a child to settle to sleep, comforting a child that is ill or responding to tears. Parents may be genuinely fearful of how they can parent without the option of feeding to provide comfort. How will a child fall asleep? How will they nap? Will it take them longer to fall asleep in the night? If the weaning was firmly child-led, it may feel like a form of rejection even if parents logically know that's not the case.

Weaning blues may even affect parents who were desperate for breastfeeding to end:

> I never actually enjoyed breastfeeding, despite doing it for so long. I was driven by my belief that breastmilk was best for my son. Literature implied that, by two, breastmilk is no longer needed, so on his second birthday we stopped. I had reduced feeds slowly from about 18 months, so we were just down to one brief morning feed a day. On his birthday we got up immediately and went to open presents and celebrate. He didn't notice. The next few days, we would get straight up and watch TV or play and have cows' milk. He completely forgot about breastmilk. I felt very down that week. Empty. I found connection hard. My breasts were sore and it was pretty miserable. After a week I was myself again and very pleased to have stopped.
>
> ~ (Anna)

Sometimes parents report a physical reaction to the end of breastfeeding:

> Shortly before Millie's fifth birthday, I suggested that for this last stretch until we weaned completely, should we just have a 'Sunday night breastfeed' and leave all the other days? She was happy with this, she was definitely starting to lose interest and had a 'take it or leave it approach' most nights. Personally, I was feeling ready to stop breastfeeding her and didn't like the 'not knowing' every night, so it felt like a nice way to wind down our breastfeeding relationship.
>
> Sadly my body had other thoughts on the matter! After the first full week of not breastfeeding (in over eight years), we then had our agreed Sunday night breastfeed. The following day I started to feel a bit sick. Within a couple of days I felt very similar to when I was pregnant with Millie, suffering from hyperemesis (severe sickness). It felt quite a cruel irony! It wasn't until I spoke to a few people that I started connecting it to the weaning process. I discovered other mothers of older children who were weaning or gradual weaning had experienced similar symptoms. One mother told me she had done a pregnancy test as the symptoms had felt so similar and she had noticed them more when she and her child cut back from feeding as opposed to stopping completely as she had with previous children.
>
> It was quite debilitating, and although I didn't experience the 'weaning blues' that I had been prepped and ready for, it did send me into feeling quite low and emotional, triggering horrible memories of the first half of Millie's pregnancy where I had been so unwell. I decided that the previous Sunday would in fact be our last feed as I couldn't bear the thought of prolonging this sickness for the next six weeks. Millie was very relaxed about it – as long as she could have the ice cream I had promised her at our planned weaning celebration! After just over a week I decided to take some prescription anti-sickness medication. I did this for a couple of days and the sickness gradually disappeared over the next week.

> Aside from the possibility of hormones at play causing this weaning sickness, I also have my own theory about it. Once I realized what was happening, it caused me to slow down, take note and honour myself and my experience of breastfeeding for nearly a decade. I had grown so used to the idea of The End, without really allowing my heart to process what that really meant. So I allowed myself some deep reflection time and space (mainly in an aromatherapy salt bath!) and just let the feelings flow. Breastfeeding my girls has been one of the most important things I have done, so saying goodbye to this stage has been very bittersweet.
>
> ~ *(Laura Walzer)*

Parenting can be looked at as 'a series of weanings'. As Glenni Lorick, IBCLC, reflects in her blog describing her unexpected weaning for medical reasons:

> Parenting really is nothing more than a series of weanings. The Merriam-Webster Dictionary has as one of its definitions for weaning 'to detach from a source of dependence'. As your child grows through various phases, your goal is to help him become increasingly independent in the healthiest way possible. You and your child will experience multiple 'weanings' from going to school or going to a friend's home to spending the night with grandparents, to going away for a week to camp, to getting a driver's license, to leaving for college. With each successive separation, you may feel a twinge of grief, but if you have given your child a firm foundation and lots of love, you can trust that it's going to be just fine, and you can allow each new parenting adventure to bring a whole new set of joys into your life! (Lorick 2014)

There is a constant process of managing a sense of loss and understanding the positivity that may ultimately come from that, and the end of breastfeeding is one of those steps. Lorick encourages parents to take a moment to reflect and she suggests writing a letter to talk about the breastfeeding relationship, the weaning experience and the reasons for weaning if it was parent-led. The parent might include some photos and then tuck them away in a memory box. This letter is as much for the parent as it is for the nursling.

When we are confident that the parent does wish to end breastfeeding, there are some basic principles that will apply in all cases. Even if a parent does need to end breastfeeding in an urgent situation, they would still ideally continue expressing for at least a few more days to gradually reduce the demand from the breast and send messages to begin the shutdown of production. When parents do end breastfeeding, we are looking to avoid engorgement which can lead to discomfort and, in some cases, mastitis. Some may wish to end breastfeeding abruptly. This may be for health reasons (perhaps in the rare cases where treatment is not compatible with continued feeding) or because emotionally they feel a drawn-out process may be more painful. As breastfeeding supporters, it may be tempting to urge against cold turkey weaning. Strategies a parent wants to use may not always feel comfortable for us but we need to centre our families with humility and not judgement. If they wish to cover their nipples in plasters/band-aids and declare milk is broken, we will support them to do so. When parents are ending breastfeeding after a longer period, they may have fewer physical symptoms and experience no engorgement at all. Sometimes, even if they follow the recommendation to take a minimum of two or three days between dropping each feed, they may still experience some fullness. This may sometimes be described as lumpiness, but these lumps can be glandular tissue at full storage capacity rather than a blocked duct or something that requires treatment. If the tenderness is localized and mastitis symptoms develop, then it may be that the process of ending breastfeeding is delayed as mastitis treatment takes place.

It is normal for a parent to continue to see evidence of milk for several weeks after the last feed. This can sometimes be upsetting, but they can be reassured that involution of breast tissue can commonly take more than a month. The urge to check if milk is still present will continue stimulation. It is not recommended to bind or compress the breast as part of the weaning process.

Prolactin inhibitors such as Cabergoline and Bromocriptine have occasionally been used to speed up the ending of milk production on rare occasions. However, side effects can be severe and include nausea, hypertension, hypotension, strokes, myocardial infarction and psychiatric disorders. Bromocriptine is considered to have greater risks than Cabergoline, and has been withdrawn for this purpose in several countries, although giving neither is normal practice (e-lactancia 2018).

A baby who is between six and 12 months old, especially one who has taken to solid food enthusiastically, may be able to avoid the use of bottles entirely and move to having formula milk in a cup (NHS 2020). After 12 months, full fat cows' milk can be given and formula is no longer necessary. Occasionally, an older child who has been breastfeeding happily may be reluctant to drink milk in another form. If water is given in a cup alongside a diet rich in dairy or equivalent products and the necessary micro-nutrients and macro-nutrients are on offer, this does not necessarily pose a problem.

Of course, breastfeeding is only partially about milk. For both the child and parent there is an emotional and relationship-building element that needs to be considered as part of the weaning process. A conscious effort to make feeding still a time for closeness, cuddling and eye contact is important.

With older children, the method 'Don't offer, don't refuse' is often suggested. However, for some toddlers and pre-schoolers, this will not bring a rapid end to breastfeeding. If breastfeeding is intertwined with sleep, the family may require more support. Removing the breastfeeding parent from the situation, and substituting other family members, may not be sensible when for the child the loss is not simply one of breastfeeding, but of the close connection with the milk producer. It can take time for an older child to learn to fall asleep and to transition between sleep cycles overnight without the breast. Parents may need support to develop new techniques which prepare a child to fall asleep comfortably. This may be close contact, singing a gentle song, the use of recorded music or white noise. Some children enthusiastically accept a transitional object such as a cuddly toy.

During the day, for young nurslings, the act of asking and the power of having their request met with love is more addictive than any milk, however tasty. Perhaps that same feeling can be substituted with a choice of book or a ten-minute activity: 'We are not going to have milk at the moment but would you like me to read you a story instead or shall we play skittles? Book or skittles?' Older children can often be distracted when a breastfeeding request appears imminent, and when breastfeeding is associated with a particular time of day or a particular chair, changing schedules even for just a few days can reduce the amount of breastfeeding that happens. Yet, as mentioned before, explicitly explaining that breastfeeding is not an option and offering another choice may be an approach that is worth exploring ahead of distraction and avoidance. If we suggest parents attempt to avoid all refusal, we are suggesting that they avoid conversations that could be beneficial. An open discussion of the refusal, a validation of any emotions that arise and a suggestion of how to move forward is likely to be more helpful than a frantic attempt to avoid the topic coming up.

Just because a parent has chosen to allow their child to self-wean with very little intervention from them, it doesn't mean they aren't in need of support. Parents may feel as though they are saying goodbye to the world of breastfeeding in itself. It may be a world where they found their team – whether in real life or online. It may be a world that gave them an identity and a value. They learnt about breastfeeding. They advocated for it. They spent their day talking to those who valued it – not least the little person who was its biggest fan. It goes without saying that they will always be part of this world of breastfeeding. We need that metaphorical village, and those who have fed their babies will support the ones who come next. Even if they don't go on to offer formal support or train as a peer supporter, they will often be the most valued members of the online parenting community.

Someone whose child is leaning more towards self-weaning may wish to know what self-weaning usually looks like. What can they expect? We do need parents to understand that self-weaning is not common before 18 months. A child who stops breastfeeding abruptly before that is usually having a nursing strike. This can happen for a number of different reasons whether in response to teething, a change in circumstances or an illness and can last for a number of days. Of course, a parent may wish a nursing strike to bring an end to breastfeeding, and that is their right to do so. Others may have mixed feelings but not feel able to hold out hope as a strike extends beyond a number of days and choose to move on reluctantly.

However, the line between what is a nursing strike and what is self-weaning is blurred. Too often, we hear the breastfeeding support community declare confidently that self-weaning can NEVER occur below 12 months or even 18 months but we have to take great care to ensure we are centring parents and families in our conversations. Who is permitted to define what constitutes self-weaning and does the precision of that definition always matter when realistically we live in a society where pure child-led weaning may not be possible? If an 11-month-old was previously breastfeeding two or three times a day, had no association between the breast and sleep and was an enthusiastic and rampant eater of solids and, one day, even the short breastfeed held no interest, is the parent 'allowed' to call that self-weaning? Or are they restricted to the definition of a nursing strike? What about a nursling who was combination feeding and breastfed alongside bottles and at nine months was no longer interested in staying on the breast beyond the initial letdown and increasingly preferred solids or cups and bottles, is that a 'natural' end to breastfeeding? Our response as professionals is likely to vary according to the feelings of the parents we are supporting. If a parent wishes to define a gentle end to breastfeeding, however it occurred, as self-weaning and is happy with the status quo, what is our motivation for imposing a restricted view of what self-weaning should look like? The assessment is more to do with previous breastfeeding behaviour than a strict age threshold. An 11-month-old who previously breastfed several times a day, took a significant proportion of their nutrition from solid food and overnight appeared to find the breast a distressing place much to the parent's dismay is a situation that requires a different approach.

Self-weaning itself is usually a gradual process. It often happens imperceptibly and it's surprisingly common for a parent to not know when the last feed was and only to look back retrospectively to realize that was the last feed. The process itself may take years and certainly months. Gradually, a child asks less, is interested in food more, rolls over and goes to sleep independently, wakes from a nap and eagerly looks for the next activity. They may go a whole day seemingly forgetting that the breast exists and then suddenly appear to remember and determinedly feed for an hour as if apologizing for ignoring an old friend. They may go a whole day without showing interest, and the next day, breastfeed more frequently. There may be feeds that appear to stick. The feed last thing at night may linger when others have long faded, and for others, it may be the feed first thing in the morning that is a favourite. It may be that as feeds become less frequent, the milk itself starts to change. Studies suggest that during gradual weaning, the milk contains proportionally more sodium and protein and lower amounts of lactose sugar. There is a description of 'weaning milk' as being more like colostrum in consistency. There may even be a case to make that weaning milk is a more appropriate source for pre-term donor milk than mature milk from parents with young babies (Garza *et al.* 1983). Older nurslings sometimes describe it as having a different taste or being less sweet. That transition may speed the process more (although it certainly doesn't motivate everyone as anyone who has 'dry nursed' a toddler in pregnancy can tell you).

Older nurslings may verbalize what is going on as breastfeeding ends. They may talk of saying goodbye to breastfeeding or announce that when they are four, they won't breastfeed any longer. Or when they no longer need a night nappy. They may make official declarations to test the waters and see how it feels, but often it is unspoken. Then one day, 24 hours passed without a breastfeed. By this stage, that doesn't mean that a parent will suffer from discomfort and engorgement, and after a gradual slowing down of breastfeeding, there is often not much a parent needs to worry about in terms of breast health. There may be a feed the next day, but perhaps not again for another two or three days. Then one day, it is a week. You can see how this often results in a parent not knowing when the last feed officially is, especially if it was a ten second 'check-in' as some assertion that the nursling still wishes to establish their right to access without a full feed. Then perhaps months or years later, when a new baby comes along, an older child may ask for some milk. Was that officially their 'last feed'?

> My daughter is just over three years 11 months at the time of writing this. I actually stopped breastfeeding her just a few days ago. I began feeling really physically and mentally uncomfortable when feeding her. It was making my skin crawl and I did not like her being latched on. These feelings led me to stop feeding her. Luckily for me I have been able to explain to my daughter that my boobs hurt, that she's so big now and has such big teeth that it hurts me sometimes. She's asked about having milk a few times so far but it's easy enough to offer her something else instead, like cow milk/soya milk in a cup, and when I tell her my breast still hurts she just wants to cuddle and kiss it which I can allow a little, so I'm not tearing her comfort away completely in one go. I've had a lot of tears about it. Feeling guilty for withdrawing it from her at my will not hers, and for not continuing to give her milk, given all of the benefits (antibodies, psychological benefits/comfort/security, nutrients). However, overall, I believe that breastfeeding in later years should be a nice experience for both parties and I believe in body autonomy. Continuing to breastfeed my daughter when I don't feel happy and comfortable with it could lead to resentment and negativity and I'd rather teach her that my body is my body and hers is hers, and I don't need to put myself in

unnecessary discomfort in order to be a good mum. I think almost four years breastfeeding is a good thing to have done and I shouldn't really feel any guilt even though it creeps in.

~ *(Carly)*

I had to end abruptly around 16 months for medical reasons. I found this extremely challenging mentally and physically – I was very upset not to be able to feed my child any more (even though I knew he didn't 'need' it from a nutritional perspective) and sad that we weren't able to end it on our own terms in a gradual way. I was also very concerned for my son's understanding of what was going on – he was old enough to ask for 'boob' and know what's going on (undoing buttons on my clothes, etc.) but not old enough to be able to explain to him why I could no longer feed him. So I was concerned that he wouldn't understand why the comfort that [had] always been available to him on demand was now removed and why I was refusing him it. We had some very difficult nights where he was crying and clawing at me and I wasn't able to let him feed (the medication I am on would be very harmful to him and I had been told that the breastfeeding was putting too much strain on my body). I couldn't find any resources to help me support him emotionally through this period – lots of advice about the physical side (cold compresses, etc.) and mental health for the mum – but nothing for the child. In the end we just kept saying 'all gone' and 'finished' but I am not sure he understood. As it happened, I was hospitalized for a few weeks and not able to see my son regularly in this time due to infection risk, so it sort of got managed on its own by the fact we were physically separated.

In terms of how the ending actually came about and how it played out – I was admitted to hospital Emergency out of the blue for heart failure. The first afternoon I was there the registrar told me in passing that 'obviously you'll need to immediately stop breastfeeding'. I'd just been told that I had a life-threatening heart condition but this was the thing that tipped me over the edge and he immediately realized his mistake and apologized that he hadn't broken the news to me in a more considered way. After I was admitted to hospital I asked to see a lactation consultant – I had given birth in the same hospital so knew they had really good IBCLCs on staff. And I was also able to speak with my own private IBCLC. But I was only able to access that support because I advocated for myself – the cardiac doctors didn't have a clue what do to with a lactating mother trying desperately to avoid mastitis (most people on the cardiac ward were male and over 70). I was allowed home for a few days after a week, and having confirmed that the medication I was on at that time was not unsafe for my son, I was able to have a few 'goodbye' feeds with my baby (against medical advice for my heart, but given I was still having to express every day to keep the mastitis away I decided that I wanted to give him the milk). This did in some ways make it harder for my son though as he thought the magic tap of mummy was back, but I needed it to be able to say goodbye. I'd also been told while I was in hospital that it was unlikely I'd be able to have another child, so for me this was saying goodbye to breastfeeding forever.

~ *(Alice)*

Mateo was four when he stopped feeding. I gently encouraged it. I had been tandem feeding for two years and I was ready for him to stop. But I didn't want to tell him that he had to stop so instead I started offering him choices. He was only feeding once a day, at bedtime, so I offered him a choice: one more chapter of your story book or a feed before bed. After a week of splitting between the two, he always chose to have more story. I thought I'd feel sad about it, but we had a good run! It felt like the right time for us both.

~ *(Becky Lopez)*

My second daughter Sasha breastfed for 28 months and then we carried on once a week for a few weeks more. I was running a breastfeeding drop-in group and as all the babies were feeding so she wanted to join. Both my girls self-weaned. Sasha was the younger one and I knew I will not be having any more children due to my age. I was very saddened by this. We both enjoyed breastfeeding very much. By the time she stopped, we were only feeding in the evening. We continued having lovely evening cuddles for very long, to be honest till now even though she is now 12. It is still our special time. I was quite emotional when we stopped. There was a feeling of grief for what would never happen again, but I was incredibly proud of what we achieved and how long we carried on. And of course, all the benefits associated with breastfeeding an older child.

~ *(Miriam Feen)*

I have breastfed my firstborn to term. It was not my intention when I started breastfeeding. I only knew of a handful of people who had breastfed at all, most of whom were doctors or dentists returning to work between six and 12 months after birth. Most of them stopped before returning to work. One dental friend didn't but she stopped soon after because she was pregnant and didn't want to tandem feed. I had no idea how to say no to my child so I didn't. I returned to work when he was 12 months old and fed him as soon as I got home after work. It was the perfect way to re-connect after many hours apart. I was pregnant the following month and again didn't know how to refuse giving him milk, so I carried on despite the aversions and pain that are common when feeding in pregnancy. He continued to feed until he was three years and 11 months old, at which point, after a big growth spurt, he stopped being able to extract the milk. It was very strange watching him unable to feed. We laughed about it and he happily accepted that the milk was just for his little sister from now on. He is five now and doesn't have any cavities.

~ *(Dentist Richa Sharma)*

Ruby and I discussed together that we would wean when she turned four. I asked her if she would like to have a special Weaning

Celebration just with me as a way of marking what felt like a very special milestone for us both. She decided she would like us to go horse-riding, so I booked a private ride through the woods together a few weeks after she finished breastfeeding. Two days after her fourth birthday we had our 'last feed'. Ruby wanted to put the boobies in a 'bye bye box' as a memento. We agreed a photo of her last feed might be better because I still needed my boobs! Then she had an extra long session (she asked if the last one could be unlimited) and finished calmly. We snuggled. I told her how proud I was of her and how much I've loved breastfeeding her.

The next day, I printed the photos and stuck them inside a card I made her and wrote to her about how special our journey had been. At bedtime, I gave her a box to be her 'bye bye box', read her the card which she put straight inside, gave her a gift – a rainbow night light – read her a new book and snuggled up listening to a new audio book that she's wanted to hear for a while.

The following few nights she accepted our new routine. She did ask for booby as we finished our story but not in a distressed way, more of a rhythm/routine she'd got into of asking. She'd always asked for more even though we'd been down to a limited feed for nearly a year. And quickly accepted we weren't doing it any more and snuggled to sleep.

She asked a couple of times for it during the day or referred to wanting it again when it was bedtime, and also asked about how come Millie gets 'so much booby'. But I didn't see any real upset, I think she was just processing it all.

A week later and she didn't even mention booby at bedtime. And now a month on, she points to my boob or says booby occasionally at bedtime. But she moves on very quickly when I remind her we don't do that and just snuggle her close or offer to stroke her back.

Bittersweet, but the right decision for us all, I think. And now the snuggle time we have at bedtime feels easier, calmer, positive and full of love.

~ *(Laura Walzer)*

Sometimes when a much older child is ending breastfeeding, their weaning may not be something that they choose. Not because the end is parent-led, but because it is biology-led. It does appear that as palates develop, teeth change and jaws and mouths grow, some nurslings struggle to maintain a latch and continue to transfer milk effectively. Far from their weaning being a choice, it can even be unexpected and distressing. In some cases, this has been reported from around the age of six or seven but it is not an area where there is research and we are talking about a small population of nurslings. Of course, just as with pregnancy, the lack of access to milk is not always a barrier to continued feeding for some. For others, it may bring a rapid end to their feeding experience.

For parents

How do you know if you are ready to instigate a weaning process? There is no easy answer to this one. Even parents who do move ahead with parent-led weaning don't necessarily possess unequivocal confidence that this is absolutely what they want to do.

One question to ask yourself is: if you had a magic wand and waving it would mean your child immediately weaned with no sadness and complete acceptance, how would that feel? Is your reaction one of overwhelming relief? Or does that feel like a loss? Do you think, 'That would be AWESOME!' Or, 'I'm not ready for that yet. There would definitely be a hole in my life.'

It can be helpful to consider in advance who your support network will be. This could be one of the most challenging experiences of your parenting life and going through it entirely on your own may make it harder. You may have a community of long-term fellow nursing parents you speak to. Sometimes your weaning allies will be found among them but this isn't true for everyone. Sometimes you may feel as though parent-led weaning is a mismatch with the aims of the group and it's hard to reconcile advocacy for continuing to feed alongside your desire to put your needs first.

Ending Breastfeeding

If you do want to stop feeding an older child, how do you go about it? Let's think about two possible children: Bob and Billie. Bob is 18 months. He is feeding on demand. This usually means feeding at least six times in 24 hours. Billie is three years old. She feeds in the morning, at bedtime and usually once during the night. Let's imagine you are feeding Bob or Billie and you want to wean.

How might you approach weaning Bob? He's feeding a lot. He feeds in the morning and at naptime. He falls asleep feeding at the beginning of the night and feeds during the night several times. He uses milk for comfort when he feels sad or shy. It's the first thing he wants when he falls over. When you sit together on the sofa, he wiggles over and lifts your shirt with a big smile on his face. He loves it all.

How long is it going to take to wean Bob? This is not something we can say with any certainty. A lot will depend on your emotional response and his emotional response to the process. For some it may be three weeks and for others three months. I think three days, based on his current feeding pattern and relationship with the breast, is unlikely.

This is clearly going to be tough and Bob may be sad but this is your choice and you will be able to make it happen with the minimum amount of upset if you are sensitive and careful. However, aiming to eradicate all forms of upset is not likely to be a helpful aim. He is allowed to be angry and disappointed and resentful and frustrated. He is allowed to have all these emotions just as much as you are allowed to stop breastfeeding. Some of this is about validating his emotions and supporting him through it. The idea that there is a no tears option is not only unrealistic but also potentially depriving him of an experience where there may be some positives. You will support him through a challenging time.

You already know this but it can be helpful to spell this out: this is not just about milk. This is about YOU. Bob is connecting with you and being as close to you as he possibly can. He is feeling safe and loved and cosy and warm. Your milk still contains immunological properties and vitamin A and protein and all the other useful things. However, Bob's feeding behaviour is about security and love and not much about vitamin A. It isn't logical to think this is about offering milk in a bottle or sippy cup instead and certainly not in response to a request to feed. That's like you asking a loved one for a hug and him giving you a sandwich. You may be a big fan of sandwiches but right then, in that context, that's a rejection.

I would also suggest that you don't offer another person instead. Does it seem entirely logical that at the moment we are pulling bits of ourselves away from our nursling, we pull our entire self away? That is not to say that you aren't entitled to support and your partner may be vital in managing this experience, but the automatic response to weaning should ideally not be that you are less available in your entirety. Bedtime is an intimate and special time for most families and all parents should feel they can have access to the experience of putting a young child to bed. When someone is ending nursing, they may step away a little, but we don't want bedtime to become a no-go zone for them. That means potential deprivation for everyone.

We need to show that you are still there and you are still very much there for connecting – just not at the nipply bits. You will still be there at bedtime when he feels scared and vulnerable. You will still be there for comfort. You will be there for him when he's going through this really tough transition of losing feeding. I hope partner/daddy is part of the bedtime process (if there is one) and able to comfort your child. Together – all three of you – you will be making new routines and patterns and developing a new parenting language. That doesn't take a night and it probably doesn't take a week. It might take a week for the 18-month-old who is only feeding a couple of times in 24 hours and falls asleep without the breast in his mouth – but that isn't Bob. For Bob, breastfeeding is almost a friend – like a separate person in itself. He is going to need some alternatives and some alternative strategies.

While it's true that this isn't simply about milk, Bob has been having quite a lot of milk which has met a lot of his nutritional demands and provided a portion of his hydration through the day. We need to look at his diet. Is Bob confidently using a cup? Would he be able to indicate if he was thirsty? Can he help himself? What will be Bob's sources of calcium, protein, vitamins and minerals and good quality fats? It might be that Bob enjoys drinking cows' milk but he also might really not. Does he eat dairy? He would ideally get around 300 ml (around 10 oz) of full-fat cows' milk a day. If he doesn't drink milk, he can eat cheese and yoghurt and you can use cream and butter in cooking. He might like a yoghurt-based fruit smoothie or a milkshake. There are other sources of calcium and other minerals like green leafy vegetables, nuts and tofu. Bob doesn't need to drink a commercial formula. Full-fat cows' milk is the recommendation. However, plenty of weaning toddlers don't go on to drink cows' milk at all and all macro- and micro-nutrients can be found elsewhere with a bit of thinking. Take a moment to reflect on what his nutritional sources will be. Do some research. He's been taking a significant portion of his calories overnight, so you will need to look at extra snacks and opportunities to offer food once that's gone.

Now it's time to look at sleep skills. This may be the most difficult aspect of the process, so we need to address it from the beginning because it could take the longest. Bob right now is using feeding from you to aid his drop-off to sleep and he's using it to transition between sleep cycles at night. As he moves between sleep cycles, he fully rouses and seeks feeding to help him move on to the next sleep cycle. Some babies need dummies re-plugged or a pat. Bob has a breast as his sleep prop. For lots of parents, this is not really something that bothers them and it can continue until it naturally fades. But if you want to wean from feeding, it's a problem for you. You can't end feeding until you have helped Bob find a new way to sleep. If we just take your milk away suddenly, it's really not very fair. This has been the way Bob has fallen asleep for a very long time. Sleep time is often when we feel the most vulnerable and when we can really get into habits. He needs help to find new strategies and new ways of falling asleep.

A useful resource for this stage can be, as mentioned earlier, *The No-Cry Sleep Solution for Toddlers and Pre-Schoolers* by Elizabeth Pantley (2005). You may already have read about her 'pull-off' method in her book aimed at babies. You would start a feed as normal but then resist the temptation to feed right to the end when your toddler is in a deep sleep and absolutely out for the count. You would use your little finger and break the latch just before they completely fall asleep. The first time, it really would only be seconds before. You want them to do the final drop-off from drowsy to deep sleep without the nipple actually being in their mouth. You are right there but the nipple access has been removed. If your nursling fully rouses at this point and searches for the breast, you may gently place your hand on their chin to see if they might still settle. If not, and they wake further, you latch them back on again and try a few moments later. Then, over several nights, you would gradually detach them earlier and earlier in the process. After a while, you may feed them and after the feed they may still pretty much be awake. It has been a gentle and slow process. They learn how to fall asleep without actually sucking. What then often starts to happen is the nursling who can do the final drop-off without you being in their mouth is less likely to rouse between sleep cycles during the night. They semi-wake (as we all do between sleep cycles at night) but feel safe about moving on to the next sleep cycle without needing their prop.

At the same time as working on the pull-off technique, you can work on introducing a different structure for bedtime. You will introduce other strategies that bring comfort at bedtime and can remain when the feeding goes. Before you even start, you could introduce a lovey – a comfort object that could become associated with sleep and bedtime. It could be cuddled between you during night-time breastfeeds. You could also think about singing a little song that is your 'bedtime song'. This is a song that you initially sing during the breastfeed, and as the breastfeed fades, it's a new part of your routine. It might happen during the final cuddle or if they appear to rouse and be looking for comfort. It's calm and soothing and – this is the important bit – you don't mind singing it every night for a while. If you are feeling very creative, choose a tune you know well and write your own lyrics about your day and your loved ones. Or choose a little poem and phrase that says, 'This is sleep time now.' As the feed ends, the song or the poem is still there. It remains consistent. It's the sign that it's sleep time now. You are still there and we're just removing the prop of the feeding. If you choose a popular poem or song, you might even find your nursling detaches to join in or fill in the missing words in the rhyming structure.

As your nursling finishes a feed more and more awake, you've got the chance to insert other things as your new 'final stage'. You could read a story. It is sometimes said that sharing a book with your toddler is more similar to breastfeeding than offering a cup or bottle of milk. You are devoting yourself to your child. You are sharing a connection. They have your attention and a cuddle. There are even some books on the process of weaning and night weaning that you might find useful. I don't mean books for you about technique but picture books for both of you that will usually have illustrations of jolly toddlers and rested mothers greeting the sunrise. *Nursies When the Sun Shines* is a classic example (Havener 2013). There are several other picture books about the end of breastfeeding, some of which you can find listed in the 'Further Resources' section. You could also make your own book. Make a photo book using one of the online photo companies about your night weaning journey. Toddlers at this age love seeing photos of themselves and their friends and family. It could just be something as simple as saying 'goodnight' to all the things he loves. You could have 'good night milk' on the last page.

The feeding moves back further. After it comes the story and the song. Then one day, perhaps feeding happens in a different room and then before bath, and one day, it gets dropped. You might go through a phase of moving the main feed before bathtime and having a tiny mini-feed at bedtime. Then the pre-bedtime feed may go and then eventually the main feed before the bath. Perhaps that night something exciting happens instead – a new toy in the bath, some ice cubes to play with. The feed is something that he will want to get out of the way to get on to the fun stuff. Some people prefer to leave the bedtime feed as the very last one that gets dropped when full weaning happens. You may have been working on daytime feeding while this whole process was going on. The point is though that we may need to start AND finish the weaning with the bedtime feed because the process of setting up a new routine could take a while.

When a nursling wakes up in the middle of the night, we can, it is hoped, develop new techniques that help them transition without needing to feed. Ideally now that we've done the pull-off, we are getting fewer night wakings but we may still see some. What else will make your toddler feel calm and safe? You may be able to use some of those techniques from bedtime. The lovey is there. You can sing your special song and use your special phrases. You may stroke and pat. You may put on a gentle piece of music or white noise. You're going to be finding your own strategies. There may be tears. It may be tempting to offer your milk because this is too difficult to manage. You have to follow your instincts. You may discover you are not ready to wean and you can cope with just one feed at night. You might decide that you are OK with a ten-second feed but then you move to other techniques. You may decide that some tears of frustration are going to have to happen because you are absolutely ready to end this stage of parenting. Try and be consistent but be kind to yourself if that's not always possible. Be kind to yourself if this doesn't always go smoothly and you feel unsure or make mistakes. Some 18-month-olds are verbal enough that they can understand that milkies are sleeping now and they will be awake in the morning – cuddles instead. In Chapter 5 on sleep, there is a further discussion of night weaning techniques that may be helpful here.

What about weaning feeds in the daytime? Once you have broken the sleep prop, the process will get easier. You sometimes hear the phrase 'Don't offer, don't refuse' used as a weaning technique. The word 'refusal' is also quite loaded when a parent may simply be suggesting a delay or negotiating a different pattern of feeding. The request and breastfeed was a way that toddler communicated with you. He asked and it happened and it was magic. It was a dialogue between you that made him feel empowered and special. Really not just about the milk. It is tempting to want to minimize the pain of refusal if it is at all possible. However, sometimes taking huge efforts to avoid an ask and a subsequent 'rejection' means you avoid developing a set of different parenting tools. Especially with older children, it may be healthier to allow a request to feed come to its natural conclusion and support them through the emotional fall-out. It may be easier to say that 'we aren't going to have milk now' rather than 'you aren't going to have milk'. You are in this together. With younger nurslings, it's going to be harder to have profound lengthy discussions that validate these feelings so we can acknowledge them and try and move forward. What other things can be asked for? Make a special box of books he can request. Make a snuggly book nest with pillows and beanbags. Instead of asking for a feed, he could lead you by the hand and ask for a 'book cuddle'. When they ask for milk, take some time to think about the essence of what they are actually asking for. Are they tired and looking for a chance to wind down? Are they feeling stressed or bored? Are they just asking for a moment where they get your undivided attention? You won't be cooking or tidying or talking to someone else or on your laptop. You are theirs. What else can meet those needs? There may need to be other ways in which they can own a moment of you, without actually nursing.

You may need to re-structure your day for a while – more time outside or at activities. Perhaps meals as a picnic if he normally asks for feed at the dinner table and climbs onto your lap. Perhaps moving the special chair where he normally asks for a feed. In the morning, it's a big hug and a scoop out of bed and a race downstairs to find the little ice cube tray full of fun snacks to avoid the morning feed. You may need to get up a little earlier for a while so you've got the energy to think ahead before he wakes and starts asking.

Some toddlers will do really well with limits. Some are starting to become fascinated by counting. If you've not managed to avoid 'the ask', how about, 'We'll have milkies for as long as it takes us to count to ten'? Count as fast or as slow as you like. You are in control. Talk about what you will be doing next. If there's a big protest at the end of a feed? 'OK, one more. Do you want "count to ten" or "count to 11"?' He is in control too.

A lot of the techniques will be the same for three-year-old Billie. She'll also need to learn how to drop off to sleep without a feed and transition between sleep cycles in another way. It's likely she'll have a much greater understanding of what's going on and you can talk about your plans together. She is also likely to be more able to explain how she is feeling and express her anger and frustration and have a better understanding when you are trying to validate and empathize with those feelings.

You may decide to use a token system. Each morning you could give her two or three (or however many) tokens and she can swap them for feeds at any time but she won't get new tokens until tomorrow. The tokens may be plastic gold coins (that one seems a bit too 'Wolf of Wall Street' for some) or perhaps little stretchy bracelets that she wears in the day and takes off each time she wants to 'buy' a feed. You are both in control. She gets to decide whether to hold on to her tokens. When she requests a feed you might talk through her decision: 'Are you sure? Because that means you only have one left for tonight. It's up to you but maybe check you're really sure.' You may well find she gains comfort from keeping that last one 'just in case' and it never gets used. Gradually there are fewer tokens given.

She would also be old enough to talk about a weaning party or special treat. We don't want too much emphasis on the 'you're a big girl now' stuff because that can sound scary. Big girls want cuddles too – but she might be ready for something new that celebrates her moving on. However, celebrations need to be carefully arranged so as not to imply that this is supposed to all be about happiness. For some nurslings, this is more of a wake than a joyful party. There can be an event that marks the end of feeding. There may even be a cake with a nipple in its centre. It can also be a time to share stories about when you said goodbye to something you loved. It's OK to talk about what's happening. This is her first intimate relationship and you are teaching important lessons about empathy and understanding. Your milkies are getting ready to stop feeding soon. We will find new ways to give cuddles and be close.

This might not be easy but you are allowed to stop. You have given such a magical gift to your child but that doesn't mean you have to continue feeding beyond a point that feels right for you. If we say parents of older nurslings are not allowed to wean, we will be frightening people of younger children who will feel stuck on a path. We do not want a world where mothers of nine-month-olds are ending breastfeeding because 'it's easier when they're younger'. Breastfeeding can continue when it's right for toddler AND parent. It can also end when it feels right. If you are involved in online breastfeeding/chestfeeding support communities, check that you are helping to create a space where parent-led weaning is not frowned upon and child-led weaning is always seen as superior. Ultimately, if we live in a world where we respect women's rights, body autonomy and the importance of consent, this extends to supporting a parent's right to feed their nursling for as long as they want to. A world which celebrates and supports a parent who chooses to feed an older child has, on the reverse of the same coin, support for parents who wish to stop (or not even feed at all). A passionate breastfeeding advocate should believe that. We may fill our brains with the evidence as to why continuing is the biological norm and supported by science, but the right for someone to have governance over their own body and someone else's access to their body is crucial.

Chapter 11

Family Stories

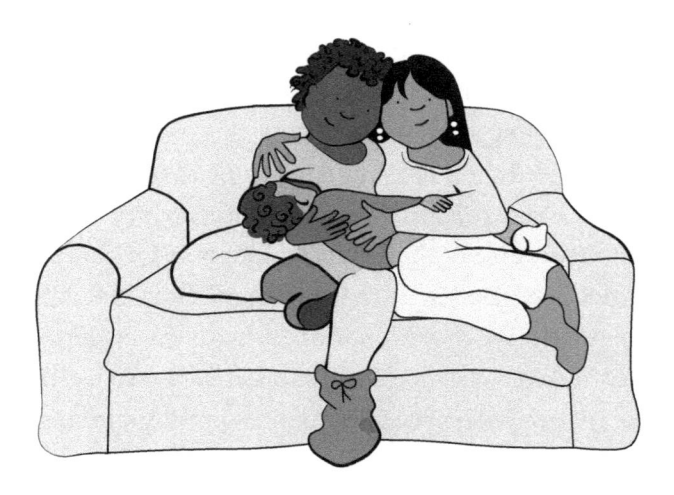

Catherine is a mother of five living in Bedfordshire, England. She is currently breastfeeding her five-year-old twins.

> I'm the youngest of four children and my mum is one of four children and my dad is one of four children. I'm not sure about my dad's family but I know my mum and her two sisters and her brother were all breastfed. My mum breastfed all four of us. I was the youngest by a lot. I'm 12 years younger than my next oldest sibling and so they will have seen me being breastfed. The older two haven't had children but my sister who is 12 years older has three children, and her youngest

is five weeks older than my eldest. She breastfed her babies because everyone in my family has breastfed. I would struggle to think of anyone on my side of the family who hasn't breastfed and I've got 11 cousins. I don't remember 'not breastfeeding' being a consideration. When I was pregnant, for the last five weeks of my pregnancy, I saw my sister breastfeeding her baby. When I came to have my babies, it wasn't really a consideration. My husband is also one of four children and his mum had breastfed all of them.

Then I had Arthur. He was two weeks late and a big baby. He was born around lunchtime and latched on and had a few sucks. I had tried for a home birth but I hadn't progressed fast enough so we'd ended up in hospital. I was in a ward with six or eight beds. I remember being woken up in the night by one of the other babies crying. One of the women from my antenatal class was at the other end of the ward and her baby wouldn't let her put him down and he wanted to feed all night. Arthur just slept. In the morning the midwife asked me how many times he had fed and I said, 'He hadn't.' So I was put on a strict scheduled four-hour feeding plan. No one actually came and helped me with how to feed him. He wouldn't open his mouth. I kept trying and hand expressing. No one told me to hand express, feed him colostrum and then try and get him to latch. My mum came to visit when he was 24 hours old and she helped me latch him. Then he started feeding. After we got home things picked up. I breastfed him until he was about 14 months, although I went back to work when he was ten months and I thought because I was going back to work three days a week, I should drop the feeds in the day. I carefully substituted each one for a snack from when he was about nine months old. He was still feeding morning and evening and perhaps overnight. Then we got down to morning and evening. The morning feed was the last one to go at about 14 months. I thought that you breastfed for a year. I remember thinking that the World Health Organization guidance of two years and beyond didn't apply to developed countries. Then I was pregnant about a month or two later.

Xanthe was born in 2010. She was born at home in the pool and latched on straight away. She fed for ten minutes every two hours, unlike Arthur who fed for 40 minutes every two hours (although Arthur did sleep for a six-hour stretch from ten days old, which I thought was awesome!). Xanthe also slept a solid block from two weeks. I was having terrible sciatica and I was referred to a physiotherapist who told me it might be because I was breastfeeding and I had too much relaxin. So I stopped breastfeeding at 51 weeks, which obviously didn't work because that's not the reason I had sciatica! I would have carried on, certainly for several months longer. I had started dropping feeds in the day in preparation for going back to work (which I did when she was very nearly one) and we were down to about two feeds. Every year on Facebook, I go past that time of year and there are the posts from when she was upset and she's crying in her cot because she's not having her bedtime feed. I look at myself back then and think, 'If only I could tell you!' I'm not a person who hangs on to anger but I feel very frustrated that I was given the wrong information. After my next child, Linnet, was born, I saw a physiotherapist who correctly identified I had no core strength and I did core exercises and my sciatica completely cleared up when she was only about two months old. It was very clear it was nothing to do with the breastfeeding.

Xanthe and Linnet have 21 months between them. I had a miscarriage before I got pregnant with Arthur and a miscarriage before Xanthe, so I thought that's what my body did, so with Linnet I thought I would start trying a bit earlier and there would be a nice two-year gap but I got pregnant first time. I gave up working when Linnet was born and took extended maternity leave for three years (I'm a Chartered Building Services Engineer). My husband Charlie had got a pay rise and we could afford for me not to go back to work. Linnet was born at home. She had a slightly traumatic birth as she got stuck on the way out and wasn't breathing straight away but the midwives did their thing by the side of the pool, and massaged her, and she was fine. Like Arthur, she was also not a keen breastfeeder. She fed a bit straight away after she was born but then I couldn't get her to feed. She didn't really feed the first night. The next morning I was there with a colostrum syringe, about to hand express, when my lovely mother-in-law arrived from Yorkshire. She held her for ten minutes and gave her back to me and she fed like a dream. Later that day, she did the same thing again – she wouldn't open her mouth to latch. My mother-in-law held her again and she fed like a dream again. Then she was fine. A magic mother-in-law!

I fed Linnet until she was 16 months. I'm not really sure why we stopped. I remember having conversations with my husband about it being weird when they could ask for it, which in retrospect is an unthoughtful comment because babies are asking from when they are born! I think there might have been an element of it being the 'socially right' time to stop. We'd got down to one feed a day which I had taken control of. They all had a cup of cows' milk at breakfast time from when they were about one. Arthur didn't really [like] cows' milk so he had plenty of yoghurt and cheese. I think I might have had in the back of my mind that it wasn't long before I wanted to try for another baby and I probably thought you had to stop breastfeeding to be able to get pregnant. There is also a time of year on Facebook where the memories come up from when I stopped Linnet's last bedtime feed and she was sad. I definitely took control. It wasn't her choice. When I had stopped breastfeeding, she would come and sit on my lap and put her hand down my cleavage. That then transferred to a little fatty lump she had on her tummy under her skin. She would put her hand on that and gently feel the lump. I wondered whether it felt like a nipple. She had a long period where you had to be careful what clothes you put her in and how you strapped her into the car. If she couldn't get to her tummy, she would scream and scream. She needed that comfort. Aged eight, she still loves to rub her tummy.

I fell pregnant with the twins as soon as we started trying about six months later. That was a bit of a shock because I had in my head that I am one of four, my husband is, my dad, my mum, my mother-in-law is one of four. Four was my obvious number. I genuinely went through all the stages of grief. I know when lots of people have twins, it's wonderful and they feel overjoyed and maybe they've struggled to get pregnant. But I don't think I'm alone. I felt really angry. This baby was going to be free. We had the pram and the Moses basket and all the clothes. I felt so angry I had to buy a new pram. I didn't really get to acceptance until they were born. Obviously, once you've got them, you wouldn't give one back. How would you choose? People did say to me, 'How are you going to feed them?' I thought, I've breastfed before and I've got two boobs and there are going to be two babies! I did get some bottles. I think my friend gave me some. When the twins were born, I forgot I had the bottles and discovered them about a year and a half later. I was very lucky as my twins were born at full term: 39 weeks and five days. I was induced. They both fed in the recovery room in the hospital. I was such a difficult customer! I had expected a home water birth again, so I really wanted to have a water birth if I possibly could. When I was 33 weeks, I sat in the hospital and wouldn't leave until I saw my named consultant. She came up between surgeries and spoke to me for half an hour. She was wonderful when I spoke to her. The same can't be said of all her registrars. She was prepared to listen. One of the registrars had told me 'no woman under her care would ever be allowed a water birth with twins' and 'I would have my babies at 38 weeks'. I pointed out this was my decision and I could listen to her informed advice but it was my call. She was adamant. Thankfully, she had a midwife helping in her clinic who stood behind her making faces at me that made me feel like I wasn't going mad. The actual consultant was very supportive. We had additional monitoring in the last couple of weeks. I laboured in the water for the first one and gave birth to Antigone outside the water. I think I was the first twin mum who had ever tried to have a water birth so I did pretty well to get as far as I got. Hopefully the next person to come along after me got a little bit further. I think their cords were cut quite quickly because they weren't long enough to stretch to my chest. I was going to get back in the water for the second baby but I didn't have time to get back in as Hebe followed hot on her sister's heels!

I was very lucky. My babies were healthy and both able to stay with me on the ward. The only negative experience was that the hospital had a policy of saying everyone had to eat in a canteen room but we weren't allowed to be with the babies. We were expected to leave them with alarms by the bed which wasn't comfortable. Luckily, my husband could visit and I did as much eating as I could when he was there. They breastfed beautifully, and the good thing about twins is that if one of them is struggling a bit more, the other one can do some of the work if you are tandem feeding. My extended maternity leave ended and I resigned from work when they were six months old, so I had no incentive to drop feeds to go back to work.

Kathryn Stagg started the Facebook group 'Breastfeeding Twins and Triplets UK' when my twins were about five or six weeks old. She knew my husband and invited me to join the group. I developed an interest in becoming a peer supporter. I became an information sponge. My friend had had twins about six weeks after me and had such awful support. The best support she had was me with no training. I was so angry about the lack of support she had had, I decided to do some training. I learned from seeing Kathryn's answers and started doing my training when the twins were about one and a quarter. I was only able to train then by leaving the twins for two and a half days so needed to wait until they were big enough to be left.

From the group, I was absorbing information about not having to stop when you got to a year. When we got to about 16 months, I remember my mum and my sister asking me when I was going to stop. There were some people round me who were distinctly uncomfortable about me continuing. It was outside their experience. It seemed weird to them. Charlie (their dad) was initially in the 'once they can ask, they are too old' camp but I told him it wasn't up to him. Now he has got used to it. We just didn't have anyone around us who had breastfed for any longer. We had one friend breastfeeding at two and we both thought it was weird. I didn't really mean to carry on breastfeeding. There just wasn't a good reason to stop and I was empowered by the knowledge that there were other people out there continuing. I knew it carried on being beneficial to the children and to me. I remember when they were about two, they went through a phase of sleeping 'perm-attached'. I was getting terrible back ache. They weren't quite big enough to hold themselves to the breast and I was having to lift them, one on each side. It was really uncomfortable and I wasn't sleeping well. But I didn't night wean them as I had no idea how to make them both not cry if they woke up in the night without waking up the whole household. So I just kept going. Then they stopped needing to be permanently attached and it got easier.

I kept going and I kept going. I had other friends who had had babies around the same time. One friend's baby had self-weaned at around one. She was a trained peer supporter and we were both very surprised by that and we knew that self-weaning rarely happens before around 18 months at the earliest, but he was very firm that he wanted a cup of milk instead. The friend who I had thought was weird carried on until her child was about four and then she stopped. My friend with the twins who had had such a rough start carried on with me. We used to go to a music class together and both sets of twins would feed after the class when they were three or four. It would be the two of us sitting there feeding our twins. Tandem feeding toddlers when you are outside the home is quite exposing, so you have to have a militant frame of mind and tell yourself to just get on with it (or get a really good scarf!). Eventually she stopped, although one of her twins would still like to be feeding and talks wistfully about it.

When Antigone was three and a half she needed surgery on her neck. She had three hospital stays during which I breastfed her. I breastfed her while they put cannulas in, after surgery. One or two of the paediatricians were surprised. I didn't have negative comments from them. I didn't have positive comments from them either. I was making positive comments about breastfeeding, and how it was helping her to cope with the discomfort and what were quite scary situations for her. One of the nurses on the children's ward did say it was good I was still breastfeeding.

I think Hebe might have self-weaned when she was about two and a half. We went through a phase at bedtime where they would choose mummy milk or hot chocolate and she often chose hot chocolate. I think if she had been a singleton, she'd probably have stopped at that point, but Antigone kept going and then Hebe got keener again and we went through a phase where she was the keener one. Now it's more balanced. Antigone did announce she was going to give up when she was six. I was suspicious someone had said something to her but she seemed firm no one had. She co-sleeps with me and asks in the night. They almost always have milk with their story at bedtime. They feed and look at the book at the same time. We started doing that to make bedtime take a bit less time when they were about two. Sometimes Charlie puts them to bed and they manage without mummy milk, but breastfeeding definitely helps them go to sleep. Hebe finds it much easier to go to sleep after milk. Antigone might wake up before I go to bed and she has milk and goes back to sleep. She might wake up when I come to bed and I'll read my book for ten minutes while she has milk and then goes back to sleep. She finds it comforting. Hebe doesn't often wake up and want milk in the night, maybe once a week. They will sometimes have milk in the morning, although the morning feed has mostly fizzled out. The lure of going downstairs to watch television is stronger than the lure of mummy milk.

I did worry when they were starting school but I don't think they have talked about breastfeeding at school, though it wouldn't surprise me if they had. The great thing about four- and five-year-olds is that they are accepting. They just take things as normal. One of the only negative experiences I had around breastfeeding was school-related.

Arthur was in Year Four and they did a concert afternoon. I had the twins, they were about two and a half. I knew they would want to feed and that would be a really good way to keep them quiet. I sat on the floor. A baby was being fed with a bottle nearby and the twins were breastfeeding. They were tandem feeding. I was a bit nervous about it but I was wearing my best breastfeeding top with slits down the sides so that there was almost nothing to see. One of the boys in Arthur's class, who is an only child, looked at me and audibly said, 'Ewww, that's disgusting!' Then turned to his friend and said, 'Look! That's disgusting!' His friend, who had twin siblings, told him to shut up because they were supposed to be being quiet. I felt really upset and had lots of feelings about wanting to say something to his parents. That sort of feeling coming out of a nine-year-old's mouth comes from home. I wanted to say something to the school. I wanted to go into the school and show them what breastfeeding was like. In the end, I moaned a lot to my friends and didn't do anything because there wasn't a good answer. I tried to take away from it that maybe the next time he saw breastfeeding, he would find it slightly less unusual.

I don't have a deadline to stop. Hebe says she will breastfeed until she dies or until she is 70,000. I will be very sad when they stop. There aren't going to be more babies. There is already one more than intended. We overshot. Although someone suggested we go for one more and then we'd have enough for an eightsome reel. But we might get twins or triplets. It will be the last bit of letting go of that part of my life. Letting the breastfeeding go will be hard. They can go on as long as they like. But probably not until they are 30!

In the 'Breastfeeding Twins and Triplets UK' group, our averages for most things related to breastfeeding are higher than the national average. Many people who get to 12 months self-identify as someone who would have stopped sooner if they hadn't been in the group. We have breastfeeding awards. We use one a lot, two regularly, three, four and five occasionally. We'll need to make a new badge when my two turn six.

I'm a teaching assistant in the reception class. We sat in the home corner playing babies the other day. We had a whole conversation about feeding your baby and resting after you've had a baby. Almost all of them told me that they had been breastfed themselves or their baby brother or sister was but they were taking a little medicine bottle from the doctor's kit and pretending it was a feeding bottle. We talked about whether it was mummy milk in the bottle. One of them did 'breastfeed' the baby. Then I told them about smashing the patriarchy but that's another story.

~ *(Catherine Wakely)*

BJ is a mother of two living in Norfolk. She is currently breastfeeding her youngest daughter.

As I write this, I have been breastfeeding for 2311 days, heading towards six and a half years. When I was first pregnant, I initially just wanted to see how breastfeeding would go; I knew little about breastfeeding or about formula, and didn't have a clue how much breastfeeding would come to matter to me. For me, the key words to describe my breastfeeding journey are: support, determination and love.

Before my first pregnancy, I had no memory of ever seeing anyone breastfeed. I knew that my mother had breastfed me for around 13 months, despite opposition from her own mother, who had formula-fed. My mother's sister then went on to breastfeed her own children for six or nine months each, inspired by my mother, but I never saw that happening. I only knew about it because I noticed my aunt's funny nursing shirts, which had buttons at a diagonal across the chest. When it came to feeding our own child, I said what many seem to: 'I'll try to breastfeed and if it doesn't work, then it's no big deal and we'll use formula. After all, most people use it, so it must be OK.' I had so little knowledge about it and the midwives used that sort of language – 'try', 'attempt', 'see how it goes' – so I got the impression that it was hard to breastfeed and not really that necessary.

I was very ill in both pregnancies with hyperemesis gravidarum. This made me feel as though my body was a failure and that it let me down; it wasn't allowing me to enjoy pregnancy or to nurture my baby the way I wanted to. Feeling this way in my first pregnancy made me determined to love and nourish my baby to the absolute best of my ability once she had arrived, in part because this would help heal my disappointment in my pregnancy and in my body. Through research, I began to understand that breastfeeding might be the way to do it. Still, I wasn't absolutely sure; the midwives didn't seem to think breastfeeding mattered that much and no one I knew talked about breastfeeding. I never saw anyone do it. When I mentioned my desire to try breastfeeding to one relative, she said, 'You'd better buy a dummy for that baby or you'll be crying in pain!' Everyone used weak words such as 'try' when it came to breastfeeding ('Sure, try it, if you want'); no one except my wife said, 'You can do this.'

In 2014, when I had my first child, Esther, I ended up with a tear. When I was having surgery in the hospital to fix the tear and was separated from my baby, the midwives pressured my wife, Fi, to give Esther formula. Fi and I had discussed breastfeeding and we had decided it was important to us, so she withstood the pressure, much to the midwives' disapproval. It's hard to feel that you're not being a good parent when you've only just become one. Then, in the first couple of weeks after we were discharged, Esther lost around 8% of her body weight. Several of the visiting midwives were quite insistent that we switch to formula. Again we declined and said that breastfeeding was important to our family and we were going to keep at it. I was even criticized because my milk came in on day five rather than day four. I was also told by one midwife that my breasts were 'too big' from engorgement and would suffocate the baby. I felt very vulnerable in those early days and weeks, and cried often. I worried I wasn't good enough, but now, looking back on it, I feel rather annoyed about the pressure we faced as well as proud and somewhat amazed that we were able to insist on continuing with breastfeeding. I understand that midwives have protocols to follow, but I felt that for the most part they were not encouraging of my breastfeeding efforts. I felt disempowered and unsupported, except by my wonderful wife. She believed in me and trusted in my body. She encouraged me to do what I felt was best.

Shortly after Esther's birth, I began to have vasospasms; this is severe pain in the breast during and after breastfeeding, and it is caused by issues with the vascular system, such as Raynaud's syndrome. Initially, no one could figure out what the problem was, though. I went to the GP, who was dismissive and told me that 'women can't have problems while breastfeeding, except for mastitis, and this isn't that'. He told me that breastfeeding can be painful and I just needed to accept it. Thankfully, the midwife who had worked with me during pregnancy suggested that I see a specialist midwife at the Norwich hospital who was also a lactation consultant. This IBCLC was very kind and helpful, and she managed to diagnose my problem and help me find solutions (keeping warm, changing my blood pressure medicine, using bamboo breast pads for extra warmth, taking multi-vitamins, and so on). This helped lessen the pain significantly and I was hugely grateful to the IBCLC because I no longer was sobbing through feeds.

Besides the vasospasms, I also had several months where I had recurrent mastitis. The pain from these two problems was excruciating at times, but thankfully I learned how to deal with them and got the help I needed. I became more determined to carry on and to succeed, despite all this.

My wife was incredibly supportive, ensuring that she made me healthy food, bringing me water, making me special treats, getting me into comfortable positions so I could rest, and encouraging me whenever I felt worried or low. People frequently, nosily asked if she was jealous of me breastfeeding or if I should express milk so she could bottle-feed the baby or other such questions, but the fact was that my wife was the person who enabled me to continue feeding. Fi was never envious or angry and she never pressured me to do anything other than what I wanted to do; she understood that she could bond with our baby in many other ways than through feeding her, and she knew that her role in helping me was absolutely vital. She put me and the baby first and never once questioned the breastfeeding relationship; this made me feel even closer to her than I had before. I'm not sure if I would have been so supportive if the situation had been the reverse!

The relationship I formed with Esther was centred on meeting her needs and loving her unconditionally, in a way that I had not felt loved or seen as a child, and one aspect of this was breastfeeding her as much as she wanted, whenever and wherever she wanted. We did this despite criticisms from some people (including relatives) or intrusive questions from others, and we breastfed around the world, in many different locations and circumstances. I decided to breastfeed Esther until she wanted to wean. This meant that I breastfed her through IVF treatment (which I did after lots of research, so I felt I was not putting her to any harm) and then through a second challenging pregnancy, when I again had hyperemesis and was confined to bed and also suffered from some breastfeeding aversion.

The IVF clinic was very clear that they expected me to wean, but I did my own research and I felt comfortable continuing to breastfeed while having treatment, because the particular drugs I needed were compatible with feeding. I also felt it was unfair to wean my child when neither of us wanted to, especially as I wasn't likely to get pregnant more easily if I weaned and I didn't see why I should prioritize an as-yet unconceived child over the beloved child I had. So my wife and I waited about a year from the time we first contacted the clinic until we felt ready to start treatment, and then we got back in touch with them. They assumed we had weaned and I did not correct that assumption. I don't usually advocate lying or omitting facts, but I felt this was about my body and my relationship with my nursling and the doctors didn't have the right to tell me to stop feeding.

During this second pregnancy, I felt like a horrible mother because I was so ill and could not engage with Esther the way I normally would. Breastfeeding helped us stay close and to strengthen our bond, and it made me feel that I was doing something right as a mother. I began to dream about tandem feeding, imagining that helping the children form their connection from the beginning in this way might help them build a strong foundation for their sibling relationship.

I gave birth to Tovah in 2018 and we have had a much easier journey, in part because I was so much more educated about breastfeeding and also because Fi and I now knew for sure how important it was, so we were resolute about it and could dismiss all unhelpful or unknowledgeable comments and suggestions. Tovah fed for the first time within a few minutes of her birth, and she and Esther shared their first tandem feed the following day.

I tandem fed the two children for many months and feeding them together helped them bond, but it also had its challenges. On a practical level, it wasn't always comfortable having a big child climbing over me and her latching skills began to weaken over time, causing me some pain. Also, I had to prioritize the baby's feeding needs over my older daughter's, which naturally caused some jealousy, and I often had to lie down to rest with the baby, while Fi and Esther were off doing crafts or reading or otherwise having fun together. Still, seeing the two girls hold hands across my chest made me feel incredibly happy.

Esther gradually began to slow down how much she fed. She began feeding just once every week or so, and then every other week, and then she eventually had her last feed when she was just over six years old. She chose a necklace made from my breastmilk as a celebration of her journey. She has also requested a photo album filled with pictures of her breastfeeding and I am currently working on this. She still feels that my chest is a safe space for her, and she loves to nestle there at night while I read to her. She sometimes misses feeding, but I try to ensure that she gets plenty of extra cuddles and special times with me.

Now I continue to feed my younger child, Tovah, who is over two years old, on demand. She has breastfed through some of the lectures or classes I have taught and during some of the meetings I have attended. I am happy to breastfeed in front of others, and I hope it might, in a small way, educate and inspire others to try breastfeeding or to support a partner with breastfeeding. For both my children, breastfeeding has been an amazing parenting tool; offering the breast has been a way of helping them feel nourished, physically and emotionally, whenever they have needed it.

I found my experiences breastfeeding so interesting and meaningful that I trained as a breastfeeding peer supporter, then as a breastfeeding counsellor, both with the ABM (Association of Breastfeeding Mothers). I now volunteer on the National Breastfeeding Helpline. I have taken all the courses towards becoming a lactation consultant as well, although not the exam yet. I have done this out of interest and not because I plan to work as a lactation consultant. Since I am an academic in literature, I am now also writing a book about the depiction of breastfeeding in literature for adults and children and I regularly write articles about breastfeeding, review books about it, and even give talks about supporting LGBTQ+ families when it comes to feeding babies and children.

Besides this, I have donated my breastmilk to several babies and even to two adults with IBS. I confess I don't enjoy pumping milk, so I rarely do this now, but when I had to pump regularly, I liked knowing that my milk would help others.

To celebrate my experiences breastfeeding my two children, I have a few pieces of breastmilk jewellery and I wear them with pride. My wife bought them for me, and I again can't emphasize enough how important she has been to me when it comes to breastfeeding (and many other things, of course).

Before we had children, I'd read many books about pregnancy, birth and parenting, but I didn't know what would be right for us as a family. All I knew for sure was that I had felt very pressured as a child and I didn't think my parents had taken my own views or feelings into account; I knew I didn't want this for my children, but I didn't quite know how to do things differently. Breastfeeding helped teach me that what I wanted most of all as a parent was to ensure that my children felt seen and accepted and cared for. I breastfed them on demand and this approach translated to other aspects of parenting; in other words, I learned to observe them, to try to understand what they need and then to meet those needs. I learned to listen and to validate and to show the children that all their feelings, thoughts and characteristics were accepted. I think breastfeeding specifically and parenting more generally has helped me become a better person, one who is more empathetic and who cares about others and the world and who tries to support others. I grew as a person by seeing how my wife supported me and also by the way breastfeeding itself shaped my interactions with our daughters.

Of course, I'm not perfect and the children may have complaints about our approach, but I feel that building a close connection to them, in large part through breastfeeding, has been the right thing to do. It has been an absolute gift, and parenting is a privilege and honour that I am so grateful for.

I can honestly say that breastfeeding my children is one of my life's biggest achievements. I am very proud of it and I am so grateful to my wife for all her support and encouragement. Our family is strong in part because of the connections we have created through breastfeeding.

~ *(BJ Woodstein)*

Fi Woodstein is BJ's wife.

> During the pregnancy of our first child we had discussed breastfeeding as a possibility worth trying, as at that stage I think we just considered it as slightly better than bottles; certainly we knew it was cheaper, but we'd decided if it didn't work out then formula was everywhere so it wouldn't be a big problem. I maintained something similar to this position for some time after Esther's birth as I didn't want to be the cause of any additional stress – and there was considerable stress around feeding over the first few months, particularly with a painful and relatively rare medical condition (vasospasms). I believed it was BJ's body that was doing the hard work and I would support any decision she made (I continue to be surprised by partners who insist that they name the baby in some bizarre ownership display after a woman has carried it for nine months and given birth to it).
>
> Because, I think, of the age of my parents (they were born in the 1920s), breastfeeding was very much the norm to them, so my brother and I were breastfed; my mum was concerned by my sister-in-law deciding to use formula for my nephews. I don't think this was particularly expressed to my sister-in-law (although I was a teenager and so it may have just bypassed me), but because I am much younger than my brother and so was still living with my parents, I, therefore, heard multiple conversations about it, which I guess was useful for me, ultimately shaping my opinion that it was something important to at least try.
>
> As the birth approached and we read more and more about babies and the accompanying topics, we gradually became more and more aware of the importance and adaptability of human milk direct from the source. Following Esther's birth, which was somewhat traumatic, we were nervous first-time parents, following nearly every instruction from any medical professional we came into contact with – although thankfully not the suggestions to quit breastfeeding

because it wasn't going smoothly. This did cause a great deal of anxiety around feeding, plus as I mentioned we eventually established that there turned out to be medical issues. We reached a lot of dead ends from some unhelpful professionals including our own GP who was adamant the only possible issue a woman could have with breastfeeding is mastitis, and it wasn't mastitis so, therefore, there was nothing wrong. Ultimately, this rather difficult journey made BJ more determined to continue, and also led her going on to train and support others during their breastfeeding journeys. Because it was hard going from the start, it maybe meant it became more treasured.

The difficulties with breastfeeding, and the support we received, eventually led my wife to learn more about it and go on to become a breastfeeding peer supporter and then a breastfeeding counsellor. This has been really interesting for me as I've gradually picked up lots of knowledge myself.

During the second pregnancy, BJ continued to breastfeed our first child, but this was not without difficulty. Because my wife had hyperemesis gravidarum she was sick every day, many times a day for the whole 9+ months – she had had this during the first pregnancy too, but of course hadn't been breastfeeding then. The constant nausea made it very challenging for her to continue feeding our older daughter, who was three by then, but she had been determined that the illness wasn't going to force her to stop feeding before they were ready. She battled through and after the birth of our second daughter was able to successfully tandem feed them for a while, which I think was a major goal for her, and I hope I was able to support her in achieving that.

For us, breastfeeding has helped keep the children healthy and provided a readily available and free, natural source of comfort whenever needed.

It is clearly more natural for children to breastfeed well into their pre-school years and potentially beyond than to be weaned at four or six months, as is implicitly suggested on the packaging of baby food. This is demonstrated by the older, more traditional cultures around the world.

It has been a kind of creeping horror to realize how manipulated much of modern culture is by formula companies. Of course, we are all heavily influenced by advertising in general in all areas of our lives, but I had the realization that such early and important stages of development have been distorted to the point that women with new babies believe that if they don't know how many millilitres of milk their baby is consuming then there is something dangerously wrong and that humankind can't exist without knowing, even though people have managed for tens of thousands of years that way.

To be a supportive partner, it is necessary to realize it is not about you. The baby's nutrition is more important than whether or not you get to hold a bottle or not. And if you're feeling left out: (1) It's quite likely you'll end up feeding them at some point anyway but early on is not the time, and (2) You can have a dramatic impact on how easy/successful your partner's breastfeeding journey might be, so step up.

You need to be encouraging and considerate.

You need to help! By getting drinks, food, etc. (and also asking what is needed!).

~ (Fi Woodstein)

Rachael lives in North London. She is breastfeeding KP who is two years and nine months.

When I went to the first meeting with my midwife, she said to me, 'Have you thought about the birth?' I said, 'I trust my body. I ran a marathon a year ago so I know my body can do great things, even when I don't think I can do mile twenty, and even if I have to walk some of it.' I viewed birth in the same way, that my body will tell me and lead me where it needs to go. I wanted to give birth at home with as little intervention as possible.

I had always gone along with the idea, perhaps it's naive, that I don't really need to read books about a routine that my baby will need to be in. There were women who'd had babies before me who told me to read certain books, and I thought, I'm not going to do that. Perhaps that meant I was under-prepared in some ways. I had no idea of the benefits of expressing colostrum before the baby's born or getting set up with a good breast pump. One of my friends was 'on it' and so organized. She had started storing any excess milk in the first few weeks so that she knew when she went back to work she would have a freezer full.

Thankfully, my body didn't fail me. I had an obstetrician because I was a 'geriatric' (being 41 at the time of birth). My baby, KP, grew what they felt was an exponential amount in the last two weeks and they were worried. They said he was big and had a big head and I'm not a big lady. This was our first rodeo. We were new parents. We were told we could have a really difficult labour and birth and we took the advice to have a planned caesarean. It was completely different to what I'd wanted but they were actually very good. We had skin-to-skin and they didn't cut the umbilical cord straight away. He was feeding well from the beginning and gaining weight well.

Early on, he did have what seemed like an allergic reaction all over his skin on his face and body. At no point, thankfully, did anyone suggest giving up breastfeeding and it never crossed my mind to because to all intents and purposes it was working really well for him. It resolved with a very gentle bathing regime and a prescribed cream to protect his skin.

Breastfeeding worked really well for our family and our lifestyle also, I could travel with him and I didn't have to worry about carrying around bottles or other stuff. We had few problems but he did have some reflux. I remember he was vomiting quite a lot at one point. We were worried that he had a bug and we took him to Accident and Emergency where we were advised to not breastfeed him and to give him rehydration salts only. Looking back with hindsight, with my knowledge of breastfeeding now, I would have politely told that nurse that wasn't something I was prepared to do or at least interrogated her about why she didn't want me to breastfeed.

I needed to go back to work when KP was six months old and I knew I would have to do one or two long days. It was important that he was able to take a bottle and I did a lot of research and found bottles that were shaped like a breast and learnt about paced bottle-feeding. I actually pulled out of a nursery place at the last minute because I didn't feel that they were fully protective of my breastfeeding and we found a childminder who supported paced bottle-feeding and using the bottles I wanted.

I did feel as though my supply was dwindling from six to 12 months. I had one friend who seemed to have super boobs and she could pump 400 ml in a moment but I knew every mother was different. This isn't a sport!

I accepted that KP would feed a lot at night because I was away from him in the day. He was in our room. He wasn't co-sleeping as such but he was very close in his cot. I had an incredible boss. I was very determined. There was no way someone was going to tell me to express sitting in a toilet. I had a senior title and I was the first person who had expressed like this at work. It became known that I was doing it and the PAs talked to each other, in the best possible way. We set up the 'boob room' with a rota system, and because the super-supportive PA's desk was outside, she kicked people out who were trying to use the room for something else. Sometimes I had a conference call going (in the days before Covid where it was easy to keep your camera off) and I sat there with one hand taking notes and one holding the pump. My boss bought us a fridge. I travelled to Paris several times as part of my job and I wasn't going to stay overnight because I wanted to get back to be with KP. I planned the day with military precision. I fed at 5 am and then caught a 7 am train. I would express in the toilet on the Eurostar train and in the Paris offices. By the time KP was two, I was on the train with a blanket over me expressing sitting in my seat.

I wasn't in a massive rush to get him on to solids. I was happy for him to take the lead. His first taste of food was an apple on the train to Paris as he often travelled with me. He'd often eat a bit of what we were eating. He liked broccoli, spinach and cheese blended together. We also batch cooked and had some things in the freezer. We didn't really put any pressure on him. I think because we felt that nutritionally he was getting what he needed from breastmilk. It allowed us to have a little bit of fun with food. Like with the birth, there was a little bit of trust there. Towards 12 months, he did sometimes have some formula if he was with my husband or with my parents. Looking back, I wonder whether we could have balanced things differently and maybe given him some more solids or some soups so he didn't need formula top-ups, but I did what felt right at the time. I didn't have any other experience to compare with.

My husband has always been supportive. He's always said that because we are breastfeeding, he's worried less, perhaps if there were days when KP ate less or because of immunological protection during the pandemic. His mum never breastfed him but he's always been a million per cent supportive. We have had to make adjustments. It does affect him too. There might be physically less space in the bed or I might be feeding KP on the sofa on a Saturday afternoon and he's doing more around the house. I might feel guilty but he'll say, 'No, you are feeding KP.' He reminds me that it's an important job.

We are in a phase at the moment where KP wants to be with me only and this can be quite testing, like if he feels daddy is entering our intimate space. It can feel like a rejection for his dad. I met with a friend the other day who isn't breastfeeding her toddler and she's going through the same experience. She had a difficult Christmas Day because her son wouldn't let her partner do anything. He tried to put their son down for a nap and ended up being whacked in the face with a toy.

That's why it's so important for mothers to talk to each other, and across the 'divisions', not just talking to parents who parent in the same way, who are breastfeeding long term or following like a super natural parenting regime. You need to talk to people who followed a structured parenting style or a different style from you, and the more you chat, the more you realize what we are all going through at the same time. Kids are going through phases of wanting to be independent but also wanting to detach at the same time. Some people associate it with breastfeeding but it's good to be reminded that's not the case.

When I look back on my own childhood, I don't feel I was often given a choice about the experience I had. I'm also quite a free-spirited person and it doesn't feel comfortable to impose my will on another individual. I have always seen and recognized KP as a person and not just a baby. He would probably prefer to still be feeding at night but that started to become untenable for me. My husband and I were doing tag team childcare during lockdown. One of us worked in the morning and one in the afternoon and we both worked at night. It was becoming really tough but I didn't want to just pull the plug. It was really important to me to explain and communicate with KP. I spent a lot of time researching. I read different books to him and spoke to a lactation consultant. I gained a lot from the 'Nourishing the Mother' online community and I did some journaling and reflecting. I didn't just want to cut KP off or impose something on him. I spoke to a friend who had made a book for her two-year-old when they were weaning. The book had pictures of their child breastfeeding and lots of positive bonding experiences with her family and at the end there was a goodbye to 'tzytzky' (their word for breasts which comes from Hebrew). It was a symbolic and heartfelt way of transitioning her child to not breastfeeding.

We were planning to go to Sri Lanka and I knew I didn't want to give up before that as breastfeeding on flights has always been such a great tool to have. It helps with earache on take-off and landing. I made a book for KP as my friend did and I toyed about it including a bye bye to 'baboo' (our word). I reflected more and decided I could cope if perhaps we started with just weaning at night. We talked about not having baboo at night any more. The last page talked about being a 'big boy'. We made a book and we left it around the house. We didn't put pressure on him to read it but he did get curious about it. I thought more about the narrative around that phrase 'big boy'. I wondered whether it was a phrase that put pressure on him to give up something that helped him to feel safe and was advised by other mothers that saying that could make a child feel under pressure to grow up. I re-strategized as the conversations I was having kept evolving. I was going to do a party to say goodbye to night-time baboo, I wanted to celebrate our breastfeeding journey and for KP to feel how special that was and to acknowledge how important it was to him; in the end, we didn't celebrate because we decided this would put too much pressure on KP to feel happy about my choice to night wean, and in reality we expected him to feel a whole range of emotions including sadness and fear, and I had prepared myself to listen to him and hold the space for those feelings as he processed them; so we had an evening with two close neighbours and a bag of balloons. It wasn't a 'party' but positive contact with adults who loved him, and his emotional cup was full as he went into that Friday night ready not to have baboo for the first time. On Saturday and Sunday, he could have the boob in the day as much as he wanted. He did wake up a couple of times in the night and I sat with him and said he was safe and I loved him and baboo would be there at 'up time'. I tried not to use the word 'not' and just focused on when baboo would happen. I said I knew it felt scary but we were here to help him. The transition felt really solid and calm. It felt reflective of his journey so far, that he was respected and spoken to like he was part of the process.

Breastfeeding has been really special for him. In his two and a half years, it's been his constant. It's helped him move neighbourhoods, move from his childminder, cope with him not seeing his grandparents. It's helped him be a brilliant traveller. It's always been there for him. It's helped him positively transition and I feel it's engendered trust. It's helped him adapt to new things like his new nursery – his teachers have been really surprised. It's like breastfeeding underlines that whatever happens he's got this rock-solid base.

I do breastfeed outside the home, on the bus and the tube even. If anyone has a problem with that, then I'm happy to have a conversation with them. They could use that energy being offended by a toddler breastfeeding instead to do something really positive like help children that don't have any food right now or build a community. Thankfully, I've never had to say that to anyone as no one seemed that bothered!

When KP was younger, I went to visit my mother-in-law and her husband. She's a wonderful woman. She hadn't breastfed and it felt like she was over-excited about having a maternal experience through KP. It felt as though she was looking for an opportunity to experience baby care again and she wanted to give a bottle. Her husband decided KP was fussy in the evening because I wasn't producing enough breastmilk and I felt real pressure to let them give a bottle of milk I'd expressed earlier (as an emergency back-up). He sat there, over a pizza, giving me all his views on breastfeeding. I felt really incensed but I also felt scared. I was in their house. My husband wasn't there (I was meant to be staying with them for support). I remember leaving the house and storming off. I couldn't get hold of my best friend or my husband. I suddenly felt this wave of rage and fury – thank God for Mother Nature. I walked back into the house and said, 'I have successfully fed my child for the last six weeks and he's doing absolutely fine and I'm his mother and you have no right to interfere or tell me how to feed my child.' As it happens, KP hadn't taken from the bottle. He just wanted boob. I went into a separate room and I closed the door and we were leaving the next day. I used the breastmilk in the bottle as a face pack. I felt like I had to really stand up for breastfeeding and it lit a fire in me and made me realize how important it was for me.

When you are a new mum, you feel vulnerable. Everyone is trying to sell you something. It comes back to trusting your body.

My husband and I have been talking about whether we'd like to have another child. I'm not sure how I feel about being pregnant and still breastfeeding. But then also if I wean, it feels like a lot of pressure to get pregnant and what if I regret weaning when KP or I am not ready? It was easy to move him into his own room. We moved house, and on the second day, he was happy to be in his own room with all the doors open. He has a double mattress on the floor in his room, so if I need to lie down with him, it's comfortable.

KP's feelings around breastfeeding are changing. When he goes to nursery, he feeds in the morning and now it's not like when I used to pick him up and he was trying to get into the sling so he could have a breastfeed. It was his way of re-connecting. Now he might say, 'Let's go and get fish and chips.' When we're home and maybe I'm making lunch and he asks, I might say, 'Can you wait five minutes because I need to finish this?', and he's fine with that. If he's twiddling, I might put my hand over my other nipple and explain it doesn't feel good for my body and that he can hold my finger instead. We communicate. He's not asking on the bus like he used to and he's slowly less interested in breastfeeding in the day. I'm thinking I'll feed through the winter. I'm in the process of asking myself a lot of questions. A friend just had a second baby and she wanted her body back before she got pregnant again. We've talked a lot about how she weaned her daughter. There are times in the day when I think I could do with trying to set a breastfeeding boundary but I know that when the time does come, it will be gentle for both of us. It's not always been easy. There have been times when I've been dog tired and working full-time and waking up five times. Sometimes it's felt insane and 'why am I

> doing this to myself?' but it has been a positive choice. I'll do some more reflecting and reach a decision that feels right for us.
>
> ~ (Rachael)

Manni is husband to Jes who breastfed their son until he was 23 months.

> I had no previous knowledge or experience of breastfeeding. All I knew was what you see in the media, like a nice image of a woman breastfeeding comfortably whilst doing something else like reading a book. I just thought it would be just as easy for my family, natural, baby would go on the boob and milk would just appear. I had no idea about things like blebs, mastitis or blocked ducts.
>
> Because of my lack of knowledge or experience, I feel like I entered my family's breastfeeding journey nonchalantly. Little did I know that there was a lot more hard work to go into it.
>
> I didn't realize the emotional connection a woman has to the child she is breastfeeding, quite naively. Then after getting so much information and watching what my wife was going through, I realized how much the hormonal changes affected her too. Our journey was hard at the beginning, I wasn't really aware of what was going to happen and how it would be. Before birth I didn't really have a strong opinion about breastfeeding, and I was happy either way. Once we had some antenatal information from the Breastfeeding Network (BfN), I realized how important breastfeeding was for my child. After this point, I felt more confident in our choice to breastfeed.
>
> When my wife first started to breastfeed, I was taken aback by how hard and emotional it all was for her. It made me feel helpless, all I could do was offer encouragement and a shoulder to cry on. As time went on and we had support from the BfN, and my wife was more comfortable, it became a regular part of our family routine.

Something that started off as difficult became an overall enjoyable and normal part of our lives.

I made sure to be part of the feeding journey, sitting with my wife whilst feeding, helping to remove blocked ducts, doing what I could to be helpful. I think that a simple act of just sitting with your partner while they are breastfeeding is such a valuable way to support someone, making them feel what they are doing is normal and that they have someone with them. Birth and becoming a new parent was a whirlwind and I realized my wife needed time, and sometimes some head space. It became my responsibility to learn about things like sterilizing the pump and how to store expressed milk. Although I did try to feed my son expressed milk with a bottle, he never really took to it and preferred the breast. I didn't necessarily take that as a bad thing, if anything it just made me realize just how much my son needed his mum.

As we became more confident as a family with feeding, venturing out and about was a whole new learning curve. Thinking about finding somewhere to sit to be able to allow a feed, it upsets me that sometimes women feel that they cannot breastfeed wherever they like and feel as though they might have to hide away at times. Whenever we did go out and about I tried to support my wife by being with her, making things as comfortable as possible. As well as sometimes challenging societal views about social breastfeeding. My wife had comments from others in our community and family circle to feed alone, away from others, or even not to breastfeed an older child. I knew my wife was very passionate about continuing to breastfeed our son and I was also happy to continue supporting her to do so. In my own home, I made guests aware that we had a breastfeeding-friendly atmosphere and that my wife would be feeding our child wherever she felt comfortable (and others if they were breastfeeding could feed wherever they felt comfortable).

My wife and I wanted to let our son wean from the breast when he was ready, we were confident that we knew what was best for our child. When he did eventually wean, again I thought it would all end quite easily. But I quickly realized that emotionally it was quite difficult for my wife, the end of such a massive journey. I really tried my best to be there for her, and support her through navigating her way through the emotions.

As I reflect on our breastfeeding journey, I think it was definitely an eye-opening experience but it really was the best thing for our family. It made me more understanding as a father and a husband, and helped my wife really bond with our son.

Breastfeeding has given us a sense of closeness, because of all those times we sat together as a family whilst my son was nursing. I feel a sense of satisfaction that my son has had the best start in life. I feel that the support that I gave my wife helped us work on the journey together and now gives us a great sense of achievement that as a family we have had a breastfeeding journey of 23 months.

It definitely gave us a chance to bond with our child and the sole responsibility of nurturing our child. I felt like I almost had a 'second-hand mother experience' by watching my wife persevere through the tough times and fight to feed. I really was rooting for her and was so proud when we got to the 'comfortable' stage and admired all of her hard work.

I feel that breastfeeding has opened the eyes of our wider family, and has made others around us more aware and accepting of breastfeeding as a normal part of family life. I think that supporting my wife feeding publicly and in a social situation has really helped to normalize it.

Breastfeeding beyond six months has been very important, just from the research alone (into the health benefits) it shows how important it has been. We had such a difficult time at the beginning that every day began to become an achievement, so getting past six months was amazing. We went through the trials and tribulations and made it to 23 months. For us it was about riding the wave as long as we could.

I think it was important that we breastfed beyond six months, because it really normalized feeding in our family/friend circle. Most didn't know much about breastfeeding, or breastfeeding older children and the continued benefits. I think as a result of the bravery of my wife our friends and siblings are more open to the concept and may be more willing to consider it as a genuine valuable option when starting their own families.

I think for my wife, it really made her stronger and more determined as a mother. She has overcome so many obstacles and has stood up to the challenge of normalizing breastfeeding that it really has made her more confident.

If I could change anything with regard to my own family's experience, if I could I would go back to one of our early outings when my wife needed to breastfeed in a shopping centre and I asked her to feed in a discreet location. Looking back on it, I didn't support my wife. Now that I've been through it I know it's a perfectly natural part of family life, it shouldn't be hidden and we shouldn't be embarrassed by it. Other people in society should be educated and aware of a completely natural and normal part of life.

I wish people weren't so immature about women feeding in public and wish that society helped mums feel more confident about it. It would be great if partners could have more education around breastfeeding and why it is so important for mums and babies, and consider being an active part of the journey.

I wish everyone could appreciate the gift that breastfeeding is for a family, and that it really is about being on your partner's team. Although your partner might be physically only able to do the feeding there is lots a partner can do to be involved and support them, it is our duty to do so. It is important to show we can, and we can be there to help. I think the role of a supportive partner is being there to do everything else around feeding, holding the baby, rocking to sleep, changing nappies so that the breastfeeding mum can find herself and collect her thoughts. I think as a supportive partner you really just

> need to listen and be there, be present in the moment. Provide moral support. Join your partner whilst they are feeding, sit with them, normalize feeding within the family rather than isolating a mum to feed on her own in a different room to others.
>
> I also wish that more mums and dads would seek out professional support for breastfeeding when they need it, it is just so important.
>
> ~ *(Manni)*

Toby is father to Nina, who is being breastfed by his wife Maira at 20 months.

> I am one of three brothers, we were all breastfed until we stopped asking for it. My older brother was two years old, my younger brother a similar age and I am told I was still breastfeeding at three and a half years old. Hats off to my mum for this, it means with the age difference she spent about seven years of her life breastfeeding.
>
> Having this in my childhood has without doubt given me a foundation and awareness of the benefits. I can remember pretty vividly being breastfed at I assume around three and a half years old. I'm not sure many people can say that. I remember the warmth and security it made me feel.
>
> Maira comes from a Brazilian Catholic large family. Maira and all her siblings were breastfed, it's just the norm in Brazil, especially in the time that Maira grew up.
>
> Whilst neither of us had any clinical knowledge of breastfeeding I assume our childhoods have had a positive impact with regard to feeding.
>
> Before Nina was born we always knew we wanted her to be breastfed for as long as possible. We researched and read lots of books,
>
> We naively assumed it would be straightforward and would be an

enjoyable experience for Maira. A beautiful way to bond with our daughter Nina and provide her with the nourishment a newborn needs. In reality we quickly found out that it is really challenging and can be emotionally and physically draining for the mother. When Maira first started breastfeeding it was immediately challenging. Maira was anxious about not having enough milk, anxious about the latch, anxious about it all. I immediately identified that my support was needed for Maira to continue breastfeeding. I would sit up with Maira through the long six-hour night feeds and calmly support when Maira felt desperate. I have to say I don't think I have the physical or mental resolve to do what mothers have to do. They are amazing!

After the first six weeks or so things began to get a lot more manageable and the feeding slightly less frequent and thankfully the marathon feeds began to decrease. There were some nights where Maira wanted to give up but with my support she was able to continue. I tried to supplement with some bottle-feeding of expressed breastmilk and the occasional bit of formula but Nina hated the bottle and wanted nothing but boob. She knows what she wants!

Nina has always been a very hungry baby and loves nothing more than being attached to a boob. She still loves it now at nearly 20 months old. I see how wonderful it is for our daughter. The connection between mother and daughter whilst feeding is beautiful to see. Even if I know how tough it is for Maira sometimes. It would be fair to say that Maira has an aversion to breastfeeding but her ability to continue through this has been incredible. She wants to continue for as long as possible even with the aversion as we both know of the benefits.

Nina now only feeds three times per day. Breakfast, lunch and dinner. She asks for boob many times a day but is at an age where you can reason with her a little and offer alternatives normally in the form of something sweet. We parent with snacks! (If anyone asks, we offer carrot sticks.) We are both so grateful for the breastfeeding support groups we were able to attend, they were probably the difference

> in it working for us or not. It's a shame that these groups are so under-funded/appreciated as they are so vital in successful breastfeeding in the longer term. I know that breastfeeding can be straightforward for some but it definitely hasn't been for us, but Maira has persevered and I am 100% sure Nina has benefited hugely from this.
>
> There is clearly some social stigma surrounding breastfeeding toddlers but this has not put us off in any way. Maira tends not to feed Nina outside any more. Normally because Nina feeds at mealtimes when we are home. I personally would like Nina to be fed for as long as she wants but I think Maira is looking at stopping by two and a half years old. I will support with Maira's choice of course. The bond between Nina and Maira is a very special one. I'm a little jealous if I'm honest. I am positive that breastfeeding has had a pivotal role in this bond.
>
> Apart from the obvious health benefits of breastmilk, the way Nina calms down and the security she feels when feeding is amazing to see. I also think that feeding for this long has given Maira a huge sense of accomplishment, the ability to overcome challenges and look at herself as a badass mother. She is badass!
>
> ~ *(Toby)*

If you are a parent reading this, it's likely you are still immersed in the world of feeding your child. You may also be supporting others. It may be hard to imagine that one day your feeding experience will be behind you and one day it may be difficult to recall. If you are going to be in a role where you support others, it may be particularly helpful for you to take a moment to record and reflect on your journey. You might also want your nursling to have a chance to record some of their thoughts and feelings. One day you may be a grandparent. One day your nursling may be a grandparent. This moment in their life will be significant and important. For you, it may well be an experience that you look back on as one of your proudest moments. It's worth taking a moment to reflect on that, long after your social media posts have faded. You might write in a journal, create some art or record some speaking. You could record a conversation between you and your nursling via audio or video.

If you are going to do some written reflections, structuring questions may help.

- What are your memories of your first feed?
- What were the most challenging aspects of your early breastfeeding experience? What helped you?
- What was a typical day like when your nursling was six months, 12 months, 18 months?
- Who supported you when your nursling was older?
- Do you recall any positive or negative experiences that particularly stand out?
- Do you have a partner or close supporter who may have some reflections they can share? How do you feel about what they have shared?
- What words does your nursling use to describe their breastfeeding experience?
- What words would you use to describe your experience/your body/yourself?
- Is there anything you wish you had done differently?
- What do you wish you could go back and say to yourself at the beginning of your experience?
- What has this experience given your family?

By the way, not all breastfeeding is noble and precious and significant. Sometimes it's boring and ordinary. Sometimes we continue to breastfeed because we're feeling lazy and it's easy and stopping feels like hard work. You may not recognize yourself in stories of resilience and struggle. Or maybe you do. There is such a variety of experience.

And take a photograph. It is astounding how many nursing families end their journey with no photographs to help them remember what was a significant and precious time. I know parents that breastfed for years and have one photo of them feeding a newborn. It may not feel important now. You don't have to share it with anyone else and you may never look at it, but give your future self an option at least.

If you live in a society where breastfeeding older children is not the norm, you have shaped the lives of those around you with every conversation and every social media post. Thank you. If you feel you may be able to offer practical support to others, consider looking into training as a peer supporter or breastfeeding counsellor. The more peer supporters who normalize breastfeeding beyond infancy, the better. If you don't have capacity for training, you may still be able to visit an antenatal class, offer a conversation with the friend of a friend or encourage someone online with a post or by sharing an image. Make ripples! Those ripples will help the parents and babies who come after you.

References

ACAS (2014) *Accommodating breastfeeding employees in the workplace.* London: ACAS. Accessed on 10/05/21 at https://archive.acas.org.uk/media/3924/Accommodating-breastfeeding-employees-in-the-workplace/pdf/Acas-guide-on-accommodating-breastfeeding-in-the-workplace.pdf.

American Academy of Family Physicians (2014) *Breastfeeding, Family Physicians Supporting (Position Paper).* AAFP. Accessed on 11/05/21 at www.aafp.org/about/policies/all/breastfeeding-position-paper.html.

American Pregnancy Association (2017) *Breastfeeding while pregnant.* Texas: APA. Accessed on 10/05/21 at https://americanpregnancy.org/healthy-pregnancy/breastfeeding/breastfeeding-while-pregnant-7269.

Amitay, E.L. and Keinan-Boker, L. (2015) 'Breastfeeding and childhood leukemia incidence: a meta-analysis and systematic review.' *Journal of the American Medical Association Pediatrics 169,* 6, e151025. doi: 10.1001/jamapediatrics.2015.1025.

Australian Government (2019) *Breastfeeding.* Canberra: Australian Government Department of Health. Accessed on 11/05/21 at www1.health.gov.au/internet/main/publishing.nsf/Content/health-pubhlth-strateg-brfeed-index.htm.

Baby Feeding Law Group (2021) *Danone Nutricia: why do they want to be your partner?* London: Baby Feeding Law Group – UK. Accessed on 10/05/21 at www.bflg-uk.org/s/BFLG-UK-Danone_Nutricia_corporate_partner_doc_Mar2021.pdf.

Barrera, C.M., Hamner, H.C., Perrine, C.G. and Scanlon, K.S. (2018) 'Timing of introduction of complementary foods to US infants, National Health and Nutrition Examination Survey 2009–2014.' *Journal of the Academy of Nutrition and Dietetics 118,* 3, 464–470. doi: https://doi.org/10.1016/j.jand.2017.10.020.

Bayyenat, S., Hashemi, S.A.G., Purbafrani, A., Saeidi, M. and Khodaee, G.H. (2014) 'The importance of breastfeeding in Holy Quran.' *International Journal of Pediatrics 2,* 4.1, 339–347. doi: 10.22038/ijp.2014.3396.

Biggs, K.V., Fidler, K.J., Shenker, N.S. and Brown, H. (2020) 'Are the doctors of the future ready to support breastfeeding? A cross-sectional study in the UK.' *International Breastfeeding Journal 15,* 46. doi: https://doi.org/10.1186/s13006-020-00290-z.

Bolton, G. with Delderfield, R. (2018) *Reflective Practice: Writing and Professional Development.* London: Sage Publishing.

Bonyata, K. (2018a) *Too much milk: sage and other herbs for decreasing milk supply.* USA: Kelly Bonyata. Accessed on 10/05/21 at https://kellymom.com/bf/can-i-breastfeed/herbs/herbs-oversupply.

Bonyata, K. (2018b) *Fenugreek seed for increasing milk supply.* USA: Kelly Bonyata. Accessed on 12/05/21 at https://kellymom.com/bf/can-i-breastfeed/herbs/fenugreek/#pregnancy.

Bonyata, K. (2018c) *Breastfeeding and fertility.* USA: Kelly Bonyata. Accessed on 12/05/21 at https://kellymom.com/ages/older-infant/fertility.

Borra, C., Iacovou, M. and Sevilla, A. (2015) 'New evidence on breastfeeding and postpartum depression: the importance of understanding women's intentions.' *Maternal and Child Health Journal 19*, 897–907. doi: https://doi.org/10.1007/s10995-014-1591-z.

Boucher, O., Julvez, J., Guxens, M., Arranz, E. *et al.* (2017) 'Association between breastfeeding duration and cognitive development, autistic traits and ADHD symptoms: a multicenter study in Spain.' *Pediatric Research 81*, 3, 434–442. doi: 10.1038/pr.2016.238.

Branger, B., Camelot, F., Droz, D., Houbiers, B. *et al.* (2019) 'Breastfeeding and early childhood caries. Review of the literature, recommendations, and prevention.' *Archives de Pédiatrie 26*, 8, 497–503.

Breastfeeding Medicine (2012) *ABM affirms breastfeeding beyond infancy as the biological norm.* Chicago: The Academy of Breastfeeding Medicine. Accessed on 01/05/21 at https://bfmed.wordpress.com/2012/05/15/abm-affirms-breastfeeding-beyond-infancy-as-the-biological-norm.

British Medical Journal (2021) 'Views and reviews: why were breastfeeding women in the UK denied the Covid-19 vaccine?' 372, n4. Accessed on 02/09/21 at www.bmj.com/content/372/bmj.n4/rapid-responses.

Brown, A. (2017) *Why Starting Solids Matters.* London: Pinter and Martin.

Brown, A. (2019) *Why Breastfeeding Grief and Trauma Matter.* London: Pinter and Martin.

Bryant, M. (2020) 'Maternity leave: US policy is worst on list of the world's richest countries.' *The Guardian*, 27 January. Accessed on 20/04/21 at www.theguardian.com/us-news/2020/jan/27/maternity-leave-us-policy-worst-worlds-richest-countries.

Cattaneo, A., Pani, P., Carletti, C., on behalf of the Follow-on Formula Research Group, *et al.* (2015) 'Advertisements of follow-on formula and their perception by pregnant women and mothers in Italy.' *Archives of Disease in Childhood 100*, 4, 323–328. doi: https://dx.doi.org/10.1136/archdischild-2014-306996.

Centers for Disease Control and Prevention (2018) *Fortified Cow's Milk and Milk Alternatives.* US Department of Health and Human Services. Accessed on 10/05/21 at www.cdc.gov/nutrition/InfantandToddlerNutrition/foods-and-drinks/cows-milk-and-milk-alternatives.html.

Cohen, R., Mrtek, M.B. and Mrtek, R.G. (1995) 'Comparison of maternal absenteeism and infant illness rates among breast-feeding and formula-feeding women in two corporations.' *American Journal of Health Promotion 10*, 2, 148–153. doi: https://doi.org/10.4278/0890-1171-10.2.148.

Constantine, Z. (2014) *UAE mothers divided over breastfeeding law.* UAE: Al Jazeera. Accessed on 11/05/21 at www.aljazeera.com/news/2014/4/22/uae-mothers-divided-over-breastfeeding-law.

Czosnykowska-Łukacka, M., Orczyk-Pawiłowicz, M., Broers, B. and Królak-Olejnik, B. (2019) 'Lactoferrin in human milk of prolonged lactation.' *Nutrients 11*, 10, 2350. doi: https://doi.org/10.3390/nu11102350.

Dallas, M.E. (2018) *Most U.S. babies start solid foods too soon.* USA: WebMD news from HealthDay. Accessed on 10/05/21 at www.webmd.com/baby/news/20180104/most-us-babies-start-solid-foods-too-soon.

Dee, D.L., Li, R., Lee, L.C. and Grummer-Strawn, L.M. (2007) 'Associations between breastfeeding practices and young children's language and motor skill development.' *Pediatrics 119*, S1, S92–S98. doi: 10.1542/peds.2006-2089N.

Dettwyler, K.A. (1995) 'A time to wean: the hominid blueprint for the natural age of weaning in modern human populations.' In P. Stuart-Macadam and K.A. Dettwyler (eds) *Breastfeeding: Biocultural Perspectives.* Piscataway, NJ: Aldine Transaction Publishing.

Dettwyler, K.A. (2015) *Court letter.* Delaware: Kathy Dettwyler. Accessed on 12/05/21 at https://kathydettwyler.weebly.com/2015-court-letter.html.

Devenish, G., Mukhtar, A., Begley, A., Spencer, A.J. *et al.* (2020) 'Early childhood feeding practices and dental caries among Australian preschoolers.' *The American Journal of Clinical Nutrition 111*, 4, 821–828. doi: 10.1093/ajcn/nqaa012.

Dewey, K.G. (2001) 'Nutrition, growth, and complementary feeding of the breastfed infant.' *Pediatric Clinics of North America 48*, 1, 87–104. doi: 10.1016/s0031-3955(05)70287-x.

Dewey, K.G., Finley, D.A. and Lönnerdal, B. (1984) 'Breast milk volume and composition during late lactation (7–20 months).' *Journal of Pediatric Gastroenterology and Nutrition 3*, 5, 713–720. doi: 10.1097/00005176-198411000-00014.

Doan, T., Gay, C.L., Kennedy, H.P., Newman, J. and Lee, K.A. (2014) 'Night-time breastfeeding behavior is associated with more nocturnal sleep among first-time mothers at one month postpartum.' *Journal of Clinical Sleep Medicine 10*, 3, 313–319. doi: https://doi.org/10.5664/jcsm.3538.

Duazo, P., Avila, J. and Kuzawa, C.W. (2010) 'Breastfeeding and later psychosocial development in the Philippines.' *American Journal of Human Biology 22*, 6, 725–730.

Duijts, L., Jaddoe, V.W.V., Hofman, A. and Moll, H.A. (2010) 'Prolonged and exclusive breastfeeding reduces the risk of infectious diseases in infancy.' *Pediatrics 126*, 1, e18–e25. doi: 10.1542/peds.2008-3256.

e-lactancia (2018) *Bromocriptine Mesilate.* Spain: APILAM (Association for Promotion of and Cultural and Scientific Research into Breastfeeding). Accessed on 12/05/21 at www.e-lactancia.org/breastfeeding/bromocriptine-mesilate/product.

Eglash, A., Simon, L., The Academy of Breastfeeding Medicine, Brodribb, W. *et al.* (2017) 'ABM Clinical Protocol #8: Human Milk Storage Information for Home Use for Full-Term Infants, Revised 2017.' *Breastfeeding Medicine 12*, 7, 390–395. doi: https://doi.org/10.1089/bfm.2017.29047.aje.

Elias, M.F., Nicolson, N.A., Bora, C. and Johnston, J. (1986) 'Sleep/wake patterns of breast-fed infants in the first 2 years of life.' *Pediatrics 77*, 3, 322–329.

Family Planning Association (2017) *Your guide to contraceptive choices – after you've had your baby.* UK: Family Planning Association (FPA). Accessed on 10/05/21 at https://www.fpa.org.uk/product/contraceptive-choices-after-youve-had-your-baby.

First Steps Nutrition Trust (2015, updated 2020) *Eating well: the first year. A guide to introducing solids and eating well up to baby's first birthday.* London: First Steps Nutrition Trust. Accessed on 10/05/21 at www.firststepsnutrition.org/eating-well-infants-new-mums.

Flower, H. (2019) *Adventures in Tandem Nursing: Breastfeeding During Pregnancy and Beyond.* 2nd edition. California: CreateSpace Independent Publishing.

Flower, H. and López, G. (2019) *New Study on Breastfeeding and Miscarriage: Cause for Concern?* La Leche League International. Accessed on 12/05/21 at www.llli.org/new-study-on-breastfeeding-and-miscarriage-cause-for-concern.

Food Standards Agency (2015) 'EAT Study: early introduction of allergenic foods to induce tolerance.' Accessed on 02/09/21 at www.food.gov.uk/research/food-allergy-and-intolerance-research/eat-study-early-introduction-of-allergenic-foods-to-induce-tolerance.

Fortune Business Insights (2020) *Infant Formula Market Size, Share and COVID-19 Impact Analysis, By Type (Infant Milk, Follow-on Milk and Others), Distribution Channel (Hypermarkets/Supermarkets, Pharmacy/Medical Stores, Specialty Stores and Others) and Regional Forecast, 2020–27.* Fortune Business Insights. Accessed on 10/05/21 at www.fortunebusinessinsights.com/industry-reports/infant-formula-market-101498.

Freed, G.L., Clark, S.J., Sorenson, J., Lohr, J.A., Cefalo, R. and Curtis, P. (1995) 'National assessment of physicians' breast-feeding knowledge, attitudes, training, and experience.' *Journal of the American Medical Association* 273, 6, 472–476.

Garza, C., Johnson, C.A., Smith, E.O. and Nichols, B.L. (1983) 'Changes in the composition of human milk during gradual weaning.' *The American Journal of Clinical Nutrition* 37, 1, 61–65. doi: https://doi.org/10.1093/ajcn/37.1.61.

Gatti, L. (2008) 'Maternal perceptions of insufficient milk supply in breastfeeding.' *Journal of Nursing Scholarship* 40, 4, 355–363. doi: 10.1111/j.1547-5069.2008.00234x.

Gordon, J. (2020) *Sleep, Changing Patterns in the Family Bed.* Jay Gordon. Accessed on 12/05/21 at www.drjaygordon.com/blog-detail/sleep-changing-patterns-in-the-family-bed.

Gunderson, E.P., Lewis, C.E., Lin, Y., Sorel, M. *et al.* (2018) 'Lactation duration and progression to diabetes in women across the childbearing years: the 30-year CARDIA Study.' *Journal of the American Medical Association Internal Medicine* 178, 3, 328–337. doi: 10.1001/jamainternmed.2017.7978.

Hale, T. and Krutsch, K. (2021) *COVID-19 vaccine in pregnancy and breastfeeding.* Texas: Infant Risk Center at Texas Tech University Health Sciences Center. Accessed on 11/02/21 at www.infantrisk.com/covid-19-vaccine-pregnancy-and-breastfeeding.

Hamosh, M., Ellis, L.A., Pollock, D.R., Henderson, T.R. and Hamosh, P. (1996) 'Breastfeeding and the working mother: effect of time and temperature of short-term storage on proteolysis, lipolysis, and bacterial growth in milk.' *Pediatrics* 97, 4, 492–498.

Hansen, K. (2016) 'Breastfeeding: a smart investment in people and in economies.' *Lancet* 387, 10017, 416. doi: 10.1016/S0140-6736(16)00012-X.

References

Harris, G. and Coulthard, H. (2016) 'Early eating behaviours and food acceptance revisited: breastfeeding and introduction of complementary foods as predictive of food acceptance.' *Current Obesity Reports* 5, 1, 113–120. doi: 10.1007/s13679-016-0202-2.

Havener, K. (2013) *Nursies When the Sun Shines: A Little Book on Nightweaning*. 2nd edition. California: Elea Press.

Henderson, J.M.T., France, K.G., Owens, J.L. and Blampied, N.M. (2010) 'Sleeping through the night: the consolidation of self-regulated sleep across the first year of life.' *Pediatrics* 126, 5, e1081–e1087. doi: https://doi.org/10.1542/peds.2010-0976.

Hicke-Roberts, A., Wennergren, G. and Hesselmar, B. (2020) 'Late introduction of solids into infants' diets may increase the risk of food allergy development.' *BMC Pediatrics* 20, 273. doi: https://doi.org/10.1186/s12887-020-02158-x.

Hookway, L. (2020) 'Breastfeeding the critically unwell child: a call to action.' *Clinical Lactation* 11, 3, 141–149. doi: 10.1891/CLINLACT-D-19-00030.

Hookway, L., Lewis, J. and Brown, A. (2021) 'The challenges of medically complex breastfed children and their families: a systematic review.' *Maternal & Child Nutrition*, e13182. doi: 10.1111/mcn.13182.

Horta, B.L., Victora, C.G. and World Health Organization (2013) *Short-term effects of breastfeeding: a systematic review on the benefits of breastfeeding on diarrhoea and pneumonia mortality*. Geneva: World Health Organization. Accessed on 04/05/21 at https://apps.who.int/iris/handle/10665/95585.

Infant Risk Center (2011) *Safe use of birth control while breastfeeding*. Texas: Infant Risk Center at Texas Tech University Health Sciences Center. Accessed on 10/05/21 at www.infantrisk.com/content/safe-use-birth-control-while-breastfeeding.

Information Services Division (2019) *Infant Feeding Statistics Scotland Financial Year 2018/19*. Information Services Division. Accessed on 04/05/21 at www.isdscotland.org/Health-Topics/Child-Health/Publications/2019-10-29/2019-10-29-Infant-Feeding-Report.pdf.

Jones, W. (2019) *Cows' Milk Protein Allergy (CMPA) and breastfeeding*. Edinburgh: The Breastfeeding Network. Accessed on 10/05/21 at www.breastfeedingnetwork.org.uk/cows-milk-protein-allergy-cmpa-and-breastfeeding.

Jones, W. (2021) *Contraception and breastfeeding*. Edinburgh: The Breastfeeding Network. Accessed on 11/05/21 at www.breastfeedingnetwork.org.uk/contraception.

Kendall-Tackett, K., Cong, Z. and Hale, T.W. (2013) 'Depression, sleep quality, and maternal well-being in postpartum women with a history of sexual assault: a comparison of breastfeeding, mixed-feeding, and formula-feeding mothers.' *Breastfeeding Medicine* 8, 1, 16–22. doi: https://doi.org/10.1089/bfm.2012.0024.

Kent, J.C., Mitoulas, L., Cox, D.B., Owens, R.A. and Hartmann, P.E. (1999) 'Breast volume and milk production during extended lactation in women.' *Experimental Physiology* 84, 2, 435–447. doi: https://doi.org/10.1111/j.1469-445X.1999.01808.x.

Kocevska, D., Rijlaarsdam, J., Ghassabian, A., Jaddoe, V.W. *et al.* (2017) 'Early childhood sleep patterns and cognitive development at age 6 years: the Generation R Study.' *Journal of Pediatric Psychology* 42, 3, 260–268.

Lorick, G. (2014) *The Grief of Weaning Before You're Ready.* Nurturing Moments. Accessed on 12/05/21 at https://anurturingmoment.blogspot.com/2014/04/the-grief-of-weaning-before-youre-ready.html.

Lullaby Trust, The (2021) *Breastfeeding and SIDS.* London: The Lullaby Trust. Accessed on 11/05/21 at www.lullabytrust.org.uk/safer-sleep-advice/breastfeeding.

Madarshahian, F. and Hassanabadi, M. (2012) 'A comparative study of breastfeeding during pregnancy: impact on maternal and newborn outcomes.' *Journal of Nursing Research 20,* 1, 74–80. doi: 10.1097/JNR.0b013e31824777c1.

Mahon-Daly, P. and Andrews, G.J. (2002) 'Liminality and breastfeeding: women negotiating space and two bodies.' *Health & Place 8,* 61–76.

Marquis, G.S., Penny, M.E., Diaz, J.M. and Marin, R.M. (2002) 'Postpartum consequences of an overlap of breastfeeding and pregnancy: reduced breast milk intake and growth during early infancy.' *Pediatrics 109,* 4, e56. doi: 10.1542/peds.109.4.e56.

Mason, F. and Greer, H. (2018) *DON'T PUSH IT: Why the formula milk industry must clean up its act.* London: The Save The Children Fund. Accessed on 10/05/21 at www.savethechildren.org.uk/content/dam/gb/reports/health/dont-push-it.pdf.

Maternity Action (2016) *Continuing to breastfeed when you return to work: Summary of Squillaci v WS Atkins (Services) Ltd.* Accessed on 01/05/21 at www.maternityaction.org.uk/wp-content/uploads/2015/05/Continuing-to-breastfeed-when-you-return-to-work-2016-1.pdf.

Matsumoto, N., Yorifuji, T., Nakamura, K., Ikeda, M., Tsukahara, H. and Doi, H. (2020) 'Breastfeeding and risk of food allergy: a nationwide birth cohort in Japan.' *Allergology International 69,* 1, 91–97. doi: https://doi.org/10.1016/j.alit.2019.08.007.

Mcfarlane and Ambacher v easyJet Airline Company Limited [2016] Bristol, cases 1401496/2015 and 3401933/2015. *Unite Legal Services.* Accessed on 01/05/21 at www.unitelegalservices.org/media/1806/mcfarlane-ambacher-v-easyjet-airline-company-limited-2016.pdf.

McKenna, J.J. (2007) *Sleeping With Your Baby: A Parents' Guide to Cosleeping.* Reprint. *Cosleeping around the world.* Indiana: The Natural Child Project. Accessed on 12/05/21 at www.naturalchild.org/articles/james_mckenna/cosleeping_world.html.

McKenna, J.J. and Gettler, L.T. (2016) 'There is no such thing as infant sleep, there is no such thing as breastfeeding, there is only breastsleeping.' *Acta Paediatrica 105,* 17–21. doi: 10.1111/apa.13161.

Mohrbacher, N. (2015) *Many Moms May Have Been Taught to Breastfeed Incorrectly: Surprising New Research.* B*E*S*T Doula Service. Accessed on 11/05/21 at https://bestdoulas.com/wp-content/uploads/2020/07/bf-nature.pdf.

Mohrbacher, N. (2020) *Milk Production and Menses: What's the Connection?* Nancy Mohrbacher. Accessed on 10/05/21 at www.nancymohrbacher.com/articles/2020/5/25/milk-production-and-menses-whats-the-connection.

Molitoris, J. (2019) 'Breastfeeding during pregnancy and the risk of miscarriage.' *Perspectives on Sexual and Reproductive Health 51,* 3, 153–163. doi: https://doi.org/10.1363/psrh.12120.

Monasta, L., Cetin, I. and Davanzo, R. (2014) 'Breastfeeding during pregnancy: safety and socioeconomic status.' *Breastfeeding Medicine 9*, 6, 322. doi: https://doi.org/10.1089/bfm.2014.0045.

Moscone, S.R. and Moore, M.J. (1993) 'Breastfeeding during pregnancy.' *Journal of Human Lactation 9*, 2, 83–88. doi: 10.1177/089033449300900219.

Moynihan, P., Tanner, L.M., Holmes, R.D., Hillier-Brown, F. *et al.* (2019) 'Systematic review of evidence pertaining to factors that modify risk of early childhood caries.' *JDR Clinical & Translational Research 4*, 3, 202–216. doi: 10.1177/2380084418824262.

Nagle, M. (2021) *Frequent Night Waking with Your Breastfed Baby – What's Normal?* Baby Chick. Accessed on 10/05/21 at www.baby-chick.com/breastfed-baby-night-waking.

Negin, J., Coffman, J., Vizintin, P. and Raynes-Greenow, C. (2016) 'The influence of grandmothers on breastfeeding rates: a systematic review.' *BMC Pregnancy and Childbirth 16*, 91. doi: https://doi.org/10.1186/s12884-016-0880-5.

Neville, M.C., Keller, R., Seacat, J., Lutes, V. *et al.* (1988) 'Studies in human lactation: milk volumes in lactating women during the onset of lactation and full lactation.' *The American Journal of Clinical Nutrition 48*, 6, 1375–1386. doi: 10.1093/ajcn/48.6.1375.

New Zealand Ministry of Health (2020) *National Breastfeeding Strategy*. Wellington: Ministry of Health. Accessed on 11/05/21 at www.health.govt.nz/our-work/life-stages/breastfeeding/national-breastfeeding-strategy-new-zealand-aotearoa-rautaki-whakamana-whangote/introduction-he-whakatakinga.

Newman, J. (2017) *Gastroenteritis in the breastfed baby*. Toronto: International Breastfeeding Centre. Accessed on 10/05/21 at https://ibconline.ca/gastroenteritis.

NHS (2018a) *Drinks and cups for babies and young children*. UK: NHS. Accessed on 10/05/21 at www.nhs.uk/conditions/baby/weaning-and-feeding/drinks-and-cups-for-babies-and-young-children.

NHS (2018b) *Neonatal herpes (herpes in a baby)*. UK: NHS. Accessed on 10/05/21 at www.nhs.uk/conditions/neonatal-herpes.

NHS (2020) *How to stop breastfeeding*. UK: NHS. Accessed on 11/05/21 at www.nhs.uk/conditions/baby/breastfeeding-and-bottle-feeding/breastfeeding/how-to-stop.

NSPCC (2021) *PANTS (the underwear rule)*. London: NSPCC. Accessed on 17/05/21 at www.nspcc.org.uk/keeping-children-safe/support-for-parents/pants-underwear-rule.

Oddy, W.H., Kendall, G.E., Li, J., Jacoby, P. *et al.* (2010) 'The long-term effects of breastfeeding on child and adolescent mental health: a pregnancy cohort study followed for 14 years.' *The Journal of Pediatrics 156*, 4, 568–574. doi: 10.1016/j.jpeds.2009.10.020.

Odom, E.C., Li, R., Scanlon, K.S., Perrine, C.G. and Grummer-Strawn, L. (2013) 'Reasons for earlier than desired cessation of breastfeeding.' *Pediatrics 131*, 3, e726–e732. doi: https://doi.org/10.1542/peds.2012-1295.

Owen, C.G., Whincup, P.H., Odoki, K., Gilg, J.A. and Cook, D.G. (2002) 'Infant feeding and blood cholesterol: a study in adolescents and a systematic review.' *Pediatrics 110*, 3, 597–608. doi: https://doi.org/10.1542/peds.110.3.597.

Pantley, E. (2005) *The No-Cry Sleep Solution for Toddlers and Pre-Schoolers: Gentle Ways to Stop Bedtime Battles and Improve Your Child's Sleep*. New York: McGraw-Hill Education.

Papoutsou, S., Savva, S.C., Hunsberger, M., Jilani, H. *et al.* (2018) 'Timing of solid food introduction and association with later childhood overweight and obesity: the IDEFICS study.' *Maternal & Child Nutrition* 14, e12471. doi: 10.1111/mcn.12471.

Parkin, D.M. (2011) '15. Cancers attributable to reproductive factors in the UK in 2010.' *British Journal of Cancer* 105, S73–S76. doi: 10.1038/bjc.2011.488.

Patelarou, E., Girvalaki, C., Brokalaki, H., Patelarou, A., Androulaki, Z. and Vardavas, C. (2012) 'Current evidence on the associations of breastfeeding, infant formula, and cow's milk introduction with type 1 diabetes mellitus: a systematic review.' *Nutrition Reviews* 70, 9, 509–519. doi: 10.1111/j.1753-4887.2012.00513.x.

Peres, K.G., Cascaes, A.M., Peres, M.A., Demarco, F.F. *et al.* (2015) 'Exclusive breastfeeding and risk of dental malocclusion.' *Pediatrics* 136, 1, e60–67. doi: https://doi.org/10.1542/peds.2014-3276.

Perkin, M.R., Logan, K., Tseng, A., Raji, B. *et al.* (2016) 'Randomized trial of introduction of allergenic foods in breast-fed infants.' *The New England Journal of Medicine* 374, 1733–1743. doi: 10.1056/NEJMoa1514210.

Perrin, M.T., Fogleman, A.D., Newburg, D.S. and Allen, J.C. (2017) 'A longitudinal study of human milk composition in the second year postpartum: implications for human milk banking.' *Maternal & Child Nutrition* 13, e12239.

Peters, S.A.E., Yang, L., Guo, Y., Chen, Y. *et al.* (2017) 'Breastfeeding and the risk of maternal cardiovascular disease: a prospective study of 300 000 Chinese women.' *Journal of the American Heart Association* 6, 6, e006081. doi: 10.1161/JAHA.117.006081.

Pinho-Gomes, A.C., Morelli, G., Jones, A. and Woodward, M. (2021) 'Association of lactation with maternal risk of type 2 diabetes – a systematic review and meta-analysis of observational studies.' *Diabetes, Obesity and Metabolism*. Online ahead of print. doi: 10.1111/dom.14417.

Pisacane, A., De Vizia, B., Valiante, A., Vaccaro, F. *et al.* (1995) 'Iron status in breast-fed infants.' *The Journal of Pediatrics* 127, 3, 429–431. doi: 10.1016/s0022-3476(95)70076-5.

Planned Parenthood (2021) *Breastfeeding.* USA: Planned Parenthood Federation of America Inc. Accessed on 10/05/21 at www.plannedparenthood.org/learn/birth-control/breastfeeding.

Price, A., Brown, J., Bittman, M., Wake, M., Quach, J. and Hiscock, H. (2014) 'Children's sleep patterns from 0 to 9 years: Australian population longitudinal study.' *Archives of Disease in Childhood* 99, 2, 119–125. doi: http://dx.doi.org/10.1136/archdischild-2013-304150.

Public Health Agency of Canada (2020) *Breastfeeding your baby.* Ottawa: Government of Canada, Public Health Agency of Canada, Health Canada. Accessed on 28/04/21 at www.canada.ca/en/public-health/services/health-promotion/childhood-adolescence/stages-childhood/infancy-birth-two-years/breastfeeding-infant-nutrition.html.

Public Health England (2019) *Guidance: Breastfeeding and Dental Health.* Public Health England. Accessed on 11/05/21 at www.gov.uk/government/publications/breastfeeding-and-dental-health/breastfeeding-and-dental-health.

Public Health England, Scientific Advisory Committee on Nutrition (2018) *Feeding in the First Year of Life: SACN Report.* Public Health England. Accessed on 10/05/21 at www.gov.uk/government/publications/feeding-in-the-first-year-of-life-sacn-report.

Regan, L. (2018a) *Miscarriage: What Every Woman Needs to Know*. London: Orion Spring.

Regan, L. (2018b) *What are Miscarriage and Preterm Labor Experts Saying?* Kellymom Parenting Breastfeeding. Accessed on 10/05/21 at https://kellymom.com/tandem-faq/02miscarriage.

Reid, N. (2020) *Anti-Racism and White Privilege Course*. Nova Reid. Accessed on 07/06/20 at https://novareid.com/asp-products/anti-racism-white-privilege-course.

Renfrew, M., McAndrew, F., Thompson, J., Fellows, L., Large, A. and Speed, M. (2011) *Infant Feeding Survey 2010*. Health and Social Care Information Centre. Accessed on 11/05/21 at https://sp.ukdataservice.ac.uk/doc/7281/mrdoc/pdf/7281_ifs-uk-2010_report.pdf.

Renfrew, M.J., Pokhrel, S., Quigley, M., McCormick, F. *et al.* (2012) *Preventing disease and saving resources: the potential contribution of increasing breastfeeding rates in the UK*. London: UNICEF UK. Accessed on 10/05/21 at www.unicef.org.uk/babyfriendly/wp-content/uploads/sites/2/2012/11/Preventing_disease_saving_resources.pdf.

Rito, A.I., Buoncristiano, M., Spinelli, A., Salanave, B. *et al.* (2019) 'Association between characteristics at birth, breastfeeding and obesity in 22 countries: the WHO European Childhood Obesity Surveillance Initiative – COSI 2015/2017.' *Obesity Facts 12*, 226–243. doi: 10.1159/000500425.

Rollins, N.C., Bhandari, N., Hajeebhoy, N., Horton, S. *et al.* (2016) 'Why invest, and what it will take to improve breastfeeding practices?' *Lancet 387*, 10017, 491–504. doi: 10.1016/S0140-6736(15)01044-2.

Sacker, A., Quigley, M.A. and Kelly, Y.J. (2006) 'Breastfeeding and developmental delay: findings from the Millennium Cohort Study.' *Pediatrics 118*, 3, e682–689. doi: 10.1542/peds.2005-3141.

Sattari, M., Levine, D., Neal, D. and Serwint, J.R. (2013) 'Personal breastfeeding behavior of physician mothers is associated with their clinical breastfeeding advocacy.' *Breastfeeding Medicine 8*, 1, 31–37. doi: https://doi.org/10.1089/bfm.2011.0148.

Schnell, A. (2013) *Breastfeeding Without Birthing: A Breastfeeding Guide for Mothers through Adoption, Surrogacy, and Other Special Circumstances*. Texas: Praeclarus Press.

Scottish Government (2018) *Scottish maternal and infant nutrition survey 2017*. Scotland: Scottish Government, Supporting Maternal and Child Wellbeing Team. Accessed on 10/05/21 at www.gov.scot/publications/scottish-maternal-infant-nutrition-survey-2017/pages/9.

Shaaban, O.M., Abbas, A.M., Abdel Hafiz, H.A., Abdelrahman, A.S., Rashwan, M. and Othman, E.R. (2015) 'Effect of pregnancy-lactation overlap on the current pregnancy outcome in women with substandard nutrition: a prospective cohort study.' *Facts, Views & Vision in ObGyn 7*, 4, 213–221.

Shenker, N.S., Perdones-Montero, A., Burke, A., Stickland, S. *et al.* (2020) 'Metabolomic and metataxonomic fingerprinting of human milk suggests compositional stability over a natural term of breastfeeding to 24 months.' *Nutrients 12*, 11, 3450. doi: https://doi.org/10.3390/nu12113450.

Silvers, K.M., Frampton, C.M., Wickens, K., Pattemore, P.K. *et al.* (2012) 'Breastfeeding protects against current asthma up to 6 years of age.' *The Journal of Pediatrics 160*, 6, 991–996.e1. doi: https://doi.org/10.1016/j.jpeds.2011.11.055.

Statista (2021) *Value of the leading baby milk brands in the United Kingdom in 2020.* London: Statista. Accessed on 11/05/21 at www.statista.com/statistics/709206/leading-baby-milk-brands-united-kingdom-uk.

Steinman, L., Doescher, M., Keppel, G.A., Pak Gorstein, S. *et al.* (2010) 'Understanding infant feeding beliefs, practices and preferred nutrition education and health provider approaches: an exploratory study with Somali mothers in the USA.' *Maternal & Child Nutrition 6,* 67–88.

Svendby, H.R., Løland, B.F., Omtvedt, M., Holmsen, S.T. and Lagerløv, P. (2016) 'Norwegian general practitioners' knowledge and beliefs about breastfeeding, and their self-rated ability as breastfeeding counsellor.' *Scandinavian Journal of Primary Health Care 34,* 2, 122–129. doi: https://doi.org/10.3109/02813432.2016.1160632.

Taveras, E.M., Li, R., Grummer-Strawn, L., Richardson, M., Marshall, R. *et al.* (2004) 'Opinions and practices of clinicians associated with continuation of exclusive breastfeeding.' *Pediatrics 113,* 4, e283–e290. doi: https://doi.org/10.1542/peds.113.4.e283.

Tham, R., Bowatte, G., Dharmage, S.C., Tan, D.J. *et al.* (2015) 'Breastfeeding and the risk of dental caries: a systematic review and meta-analysis.' *Acta Paediatrica 104,* S467, 62–84. doi: https://doi.org/10.1111/apa.13118.

Thompson, A.J., Topping, A.E. and Jones, L.L. (2020) '"Surely you're not still breastfeeding": a qualitative exploration of women's experiences of breastfeeding beyond infancy in the UK.' *BMJ Open 10,* 5, e035199. doi: 10.1136/bmjopen-2019-035199.

UNICEF UK Baby Friendly Initiative (2018) *Breastfeeding Assessment Tools.* London: UNICEF UK. Accessed on 10/05/21 at www.unicef.org.uk/babyfriendly/baby-friendly-resources/implementing-standards-resources/breastfeeding-assessment-tools.

UNICEF UK Baby Friendly Initiative (2021a) *Breastfeeding in the UK.* London: UNICEF UK. Accessed on 11/05/21 at www.unicef.org.uk/babyfriendly/about/breastfeeding-in-the-uk.

UNICEF UK Baby Friendly Initiative (2021b) *Research on brain and cognitive development.* London: UNICEF UK. Accessed on 13/05/21 at www.unicef.org.uk/babyfriendly/news-and-research/baby-friendly-research/infant-health-research/infant-health-research-brain-and-cognitive-development.

Velez, M. (2013) '"Breastfeeding is not just for newborns" ad helps normalize extended breastfeeding.' *Huffington Post.* Accessed on 10/05/21 at www.huffingtonpost.co.uk/entry/breastfeeding-ad_n_4117270.

Vestergaard, M., Obel, C., Henriksen, T.B., Sørensen, H.T., Skajaa, E. and Ostergaard, J. (1999) 'Duration of breastfeeding and developmental milestones during the latter half of infancy.' *Acta Paediatrica 88,* 12, 1327–1332. doi: 10.1080/080352599750030022.

Walker, M. (2013) 'Are there any cures for sore nipples?' *Clinical Lactation 4,* 3, 106–115.

Wallace, L.M. and Kosmala-Anderson, J. (2006) 'A training needs survey of doctors' breastfeeding support skills in England.' *Maternal and Child Nutrition 2,* 4, 217–231.

Wiessinger, D. (1996) 'Watch your language!' *Journal of Human Lactation 12,* 1, 1–4.

Wiessinger, D., West, D. and Pitman, T. (2010) *The Womanly Art of Breastfeeding.* London: Pinter and Martin.

World Breastfeeding Trends Initiative (2016) *World Breastfeeding Trends Initiative UK Report 2016.* London: WBTi. Accessed on 11/05/21 at https://ukbreastfeedingtrends.files.wordpress.com/2017/03/wbti-uk-report-2016-part-1-14-2-17.pdf.

World Health Organization (1981) *International Code of Marketing of Breast-milk Substitutes.* Geneva: WHO. Accessed on 07/06/21 at www.who.int/nutrition/publications/code_english.pdf.

World Health Organization, UNICEF (2003) *Global strategy for infant and young child feeding.* Geneva: WHO. Accessed on 07/06/21 at www.who.int/nutrition/topics/global_strategy/en.

Yate, Z. (2020) *When Breastfeeding Sucks: What You Need to Know About Nursing Aversion and Agitation.* London: Pinter and Martin.

Further Resources

Association of Breastfeeding Mothers (2019) Resources for schools. *Breastfeeding: More Than Milk*. Accessed 23/06/21 at https://abm.me.uk/resources-for-schools.
  These resources can be used with young people at home or in educational settings to help normalize breastfeeding.
Bengson, D. (2000) *How Weaning Happens*. Illinois: La Leche League International.
Brown, A. (2018) *The Positive Breastfeeding Book: Everything You Need to Feed Your Baby with Confidence*. London: Pinter and Martin.
Brown, A. (2019) *Informed is Best: How to Spot Fake News about Your Pregnancy, Birth and Baby*. London: Pinter and Martin.
Bumgarner, N.J. (2000) *Mothering Your Nursing Toddler*. 3rd edition. Illinois: La Leche League International.
Calaf, M. (2011) *You, Me and the Breast*. London: Pinter and Martin.
Davis, N. (2021) 'When it's time to let go...stories of weaning' (Lecture). GOLD Lactation Conference. www.goldlearning.com. 13 April.
De Visscher, M. (2020) *Bye-Bye Mommy's Milk: A Step by Step Weaning Guide for Mom and Child*. Turkey: Kütüphaneler ve Yayımlar Genel Müdürlüğü.
Dillemuth, J. (2017) *Loving Comfort: A Toddler Weaning Story*. USA: Julie Dillemuth.
Dow, N. (2019) *Breastfeeding Beyond Infancy: A Guide for GPs*. Bedford, UK: Association of Breastfeeding Mothers. Accessed on 13/08/21 at https://abm.me.uk/wp-content/uploads/GP-Guide-Breastfeeding-beyond-infancy.pdf.
  This resource written by Dr Naomi Dow (with support from Dr Victoria Thomas and myself) is aimed at family doctors/GPs who may be unfamiliar with supporting breastfeeding beyond infancy. It is an excellent summary to share with health professionals of all types.
Dowling, S., Pontin, D. and Boyer, K. (2018) *Social Experiences of Breastfeeding: Building Bridges Between Research, Policy and Practice*. Bristol: Policy Press.
Elder, J. (2019) *My Milk Will Go, Our Love Will Grow: A Book for Weaning*. USA: Heart Words Press.
Hookway, L. (2018) *Holistic Sleep Coaching: Gentle Alternatives to Sleep Training for Health and Childcare Professionals*. Texas: Praeclarus Press.
Hookway, L. (2020) *Let's Talk About Your New Family's Sleep*. London: Pinter and Martin.

Hookway, L. (2021) *Still Awake: Responsive Sleep Tools for Toddlers to Tweens*. London: Pinter and Martin.

Lanoue, W. (2017) *A Loving Weaning: How to Move Forward Together*. Texas: Praeclarus Press.

Mohrbacher, N. (2020) *Breastfeeding Answers: A Guide for Helping Families*. 2nd edition. Illinois: Nancy Mohrbacher Solutions.

Pickett, E. (2019) *The Breast Book: A Puberty Guide with a Difference – It's the When, Why and How of Breasts*. London: Pinter and Martin.
I wrote this book as a guide for young people getting breasts for the first time. The sections on breastfeeding are useful as a basis for family discussion at any age.

Rapley, G. and Murkett, T. (2019) *Baby-Led Weaning: The Essential Guide*. New York: The Experiment.

Susan, M. (2018) *A Time to Wean*. USA: Corolishine Books.

Subject Index

adopted children 169–70
allergies
   first signs of 90–1
   introducing allergens 77, 82
   prevention 90–1
asthma risk 33
attachment adjustment 152
autistic children 200
autistic parents 144
aversion (breastfeeding) 142–4, 185, 263

baby-led weaning *see* child-led weaning
behaviour at the breast *see*
   nursing manners
benefits of breastfeeding
   baby's health 31–4, 75
   mental health (child's) 38–9
   mental health (parent's) 34
   parental health 33–4, 75
biting 152–6
blebs 159
blocked ducts 159
body autonomy 134
bottle-feeding
   not a substitute/equivalent
     experience 52–3, 224
   paced bottle-feeding 252
   required for parent to return
     to work? 114–5
'breast is best' phrase 34–5
breast pumps 125–6
breastfeeding aversion 142–4, 185, 263
breastfeeding clothes 173–4

'Breastfeeding for Doctors' group 16, 19
breastfeeding drop-ins 205
'Breastfeeding Twins and Triplets
   UK' group 237, 240–1
breastmilk seen as disgusting 23
Bromocriptine 213

Cabergoline 213
calcium supplements 157
cancer (childhood) 32
cardio-vascular disease 33
chairs (nursing) 150
chicken pox 158
child-led weaning
   nursing strike mistaken for 160, 215
   overview 83–4, 205
   signs of 216–7
childhood cancers 32
clomid 194
clothes (breastfeeding) 173–4
cold sores 158
colostrum
   for newborn (while tandem
     feeding) 186
   produced during pregnancy 182
commemorating breastfeeding
   and weaning 203–4, 212, 221,
   227, 230, 254, 255, 264–6
contraception
   breastfeeding as 189–90
   hormonal 162–3, 183, 190
   lactational amenorrhoea method 162
controlled crying 99, 108

Subject Index

Covid-19
   lockdown impact 55-6, 135-6
   vaccinations 18-9
cows' milk
   never using 91-2, 225
   protein allergy 90-2
cultural influences 42-6
cup-feeding 115
cushions 172

decision-making (changes over time) 45-6, 147-8
dental health 33, 63-70
   see also teeth
developing countries (assumptions about) 36-7
diabetes risk
   baby 33
   parent 33-4
diarrhoea 31-2, 164
disgust (provoked feeling of) 23
'don't offer, don't refuse' 141, 213
drop-ins 205
duration of feed 153-4, 174

ear infections 32
EAT (Enquiring About Tolerance) study 77
economic impact 4
educational attainment 32
ending breastfeeding
   abrupt endings 212
   anger (child's) 202, 223
   because of change in teeth/palate etc. 222
   challenges during 200-2
   changing bedtime routine when 226-7
   'don't offer, don't refuse' method 141, 213
   emotional responses to 206-9
   evidence of milk after 212-3
   false assumptions about 202
   guilt about 217-8
   huge variety of ways 199-200
   just after new baby arrives 187-8
   for medical treatment 206
   nutritional needs after breastfeeding 224-5
   offering a substitute 224
   as opportunity to support child 202-3
   'parent-led weaning' discussions 201-2
   parental readiness for 222-3
   parents' stories 217-21
   physical reaction to 210-1
   picture books about 227
   preparing the child for 203
   professionals' input 202
   prolactin inhibitors 213
   re-structuring the day 229
   setting limits for child 229
   support network for 222
   token system 230
   unhappy ending 15
   verbalizing by child about 216
   when feeding is linked with sleep 213-4, 225-8
   see also child-led weaning
energy requirements 88
environmental benefits 34

family stories 232-66
family (wider)
   attitude of 50, 55-6, 59, 256-7, 260-1
   grandparents 56-9
fatty milk 153-4, 174
fertility awareness methods 190
fertility treatment 191-6, 244
fertility while breastfeeding 190-1
finger-feeding 114-5
follow-on formula
   health professionals' advice about 43
   industry growth 42
   message given out by industry 43, 250
   on social media 43-4
formula
   pressure to give after birth 242
   see also follow-on formula

galactagogues 163, 184
GPIFN (GP Infant Feeding Network) 19
grandparents 56-9
gravity and positioning 149
guilt 107, 122, 217-8

habit-stacking 98-9
hand, foot and mouth disease 158-9
health benefits *see* benefits of breastfeeding

health professionals
   attitude of 60–1, 236
   challenges when working
      with other 71–4
   disapproval from 242–3
   effect of their personal experience 12–7
   gaps in the education of 16–8, 61–2
   lack of confidence of 18, 22
   lying to 13
herbal galactagogues 163, 184
HIFN (Hospital Infant Feeding
    Network) 19
hormonal contraception 162–3, 183, 190
hyperemesis gravidarum 185

identity (breastfeeding as part
   of parent's) 214–5
ill children 164–7
immunological properties 41–2
impetigo 158
IQ score 32
iron levels 80–1
Islam view on breastfeeding 45, 170
IVF treatment 191–6, 244

jealousy of newborn 187–8
judgement 21
justification (feeling required
    to provide) 35–7

lactation cookies 163
lactational amenorrhoea method
   (birth control) 162
language development 39
language used
   issues around 34–5
   prejudices revealed through
     choice of 37
   terminology 10, 27–8
latching problems 174
letrozole 194
leukemia 32
liminality 13–4
limit setting see nursing manners
lockdown impact 55–6, 135–6
'loss' of nutritional benefits 39–40

magnesium supplements 157
manners see nursing manners
mastitis 159, 212–3, 243
maternity leave 111–2
medically complex children 165–7
medication
   breastfeeding and 18–9
   ending breastfeeding to take 206
   fertility drugs 194
menstrual cycle 157–8, 190–1
mental health
   child 38–9
   parent 34
metformin 194
milk blisters 159
milk supply
   concerns about 161–4
   fertility medications and 196
   hormonal contraception and 162–3, 190
   while pregnant 182–4
miscarriage risk 178–81
Muslim view on breastfeeding 45, 170

naps 97
natural family planning methods 190
newborn
   benefits to older child from 189
   colostrum for 186
   ending breastfeeding older child 187–8
   jealousy 187–8
   older child resuming
     breastfeeding again 188
   swapping sides with older child 186
   tandem feeding 186–8
night weaning 103–8
nipples
   infection 157–8
   nipple twiddling 133–4
   sensitivity of 156–7
   sore 148, 156, 184
   vasospasm 151, 243
'norm' (breastfeeding as
    physiological) 49
'Nourishing the Mother' online
    community 254
nursing chairs 150
nursing manners
   biting 152–6
   establishing boundaries around 135–8

Subject Index

nipple twiddling 133–4
overview 131–3
parents' stories 138–40
strategies to help with 136–8, 141–2
nursing strikes 159–61, 215
nutrition
  after ending breastfeeding 224–5
  increases in second year milk 41–2
  myth that 'lost' with later breastfeeding 39–40

obesity risk 32, 82

paced bottle-feeding 252
'Pantley pull-off' 104, 225–6
parent-led weaning
  criticism of 204
  difficult to discuss 201–2, 204–5
parental separation 167–9
partner
  support from 50–4, 244, 250, 253, 261–2
  a viewpoint of 258–64
perceived insufficient milk (PIM) supply 161–4
positioning issues 148–51, 171–3
post-partum depression 34
pregnancy, breastfeeding during
  child-led weaning during 182
  miscarriage risk 178–81
  myths around 177
  nutritional impact 181–2
  research into 177–9
  sore nipples 184
  worries about 176–7
pregnancy tests 191
progesterone (during next pregnancy) 183
prolactin 183
public (feeding in) 256, 261
pull-off technique 104, 225–6
pumping 125–6

Raynaud's syndrome 151
reclined positions 150
recommendations (government/NGOs) 28, 36, 37–8, 76–7
reflective practice 23–4
refusing to breastfeed (is okay) 136, 141, 144, 214, 228–9

rehydration 164
relationships *see* family (wider); partner
respiratory infection 32
responsive parenting 42, 57–8
reverse cycling 116
right to stop breastfeeding 231
risks of not breastfeeding (discussions around) 31
  see also benefits of breastfeeding
rugby hold/football hold 150

sage (to reduce milk supply) 164
saliva production 156
school
  other children's attitude 239–40
  starting 58
'sealioning' 36–7
self-weaning *see* child-led weaning
separated parents 167–9
sexual view of breasts 19–20
six months (getting to)
  acknowledging as an achievement 30–1
  statistics 29
sleep
  average sleep needs 96–7
  'breastsleeping' as biological norm 94–5
  ending breastfeeding as response to sleep issue 102–4
  ending breastfeeding when it is linked to sleep 213–4, 225–8
  feeding back to sleep 98–9
  fragmentation vs deprivation 96–7
  frequent waking advice 97–8
  naps 97
  night waking (when breastfeeding has ended) 228
  night weaning 103–8
  'perm-attachment' 238
  questions to ask a supporting professional 108–9
  sleep training methods 99–100, 108
  variation in children's sleeping patterns 93, 100–2
  waking to breastfeed 93–4, 97
slurping 171
social development (impact on) 38
social media influence 43–4

social support (dropping away over time) 49
solid foods
　adventurousness of breastfed babies 84–5
　and allergies 81–2
　being told to cut back on breastfeeding 89–90
　child-led weaning 83–4
　complex feelings about introducing 79–80
　concerns about quantities 87–9
　delaying the introduction of 78
　EAT (Enquiring About Tolerance) study 77
　energy balance with milk 83
　energy requirements and 88
　natural adjustment of milk intake 85–6
　signs of readiness 78
　six month recommendations 76–8
sore nipples 148, 156, 184
speech development 39
Start4Life (on Facebook) 43
statistics/prevalence 112
storing expressed milk 115, 121, 126
suction 171
Sudden Infant Death Syndrome 32
supervision 24
supplementary feeding system 184
supply *see* milk supply
syringe-feeding 114–5

tandem feeding 186–8
teeth
　biting 152–6
　dental health 33, 63–70
　loss of milk teeth 152
terminology 10, 27–8
thrush 157–8
Time magazine cover 22
token system
　for nursing manners 138
　when ending breastfeeding 230

training of health professionals 61–2
twins 236–7

unconscious bias 25
unwell children 164–7

vasospasm 151, 243
viruses 158–9
vomiting/diarrhoea 31–2, 164

weaning
　'average age' of 40
　comparison studies 41
　confusion around term 205
　definition 211
　parenting as a series of 211–2
　see also child-led weaning; ending breastfeeding; night weaning
'weaning blues' 206–9
weaning celebration 203–4, 212, 221, 230, 254, 255
'weaning milk' 216
W.E.I.R.D. countries 10
work, returning to
　bottle use 114–5
　employer's responsibilities 117–9, 124–5, 129
　frequency of expressing 116–7
　guilt about 122
　maternity leave 111–2
　milk quantities required for 113–4
　parents' stories 119–23, 127–30, 252–3
　preparation for 119
　pumping 125–6
　reverse cycling 116
　storing expressed milk 115, 121, 126
　strategies to help with 123–7

zinc levels 80

Author Index

ACAS 117
American Academy of Family
    Physicians 38, 189, 190
American Academy of Pediatrics 37
American Pregnancy Association 181
Amitay, E.L. 32
Andrews, G.J. 23
Australian Government 38
Avila, J. 38

Baby Feeding Law Group 43
Barrera, C.M. 78
Bayyenat, S. 45
Biggs, K.V. 17
Bolton, G. 24
Bonyata, K. 164, 184, 190
Borra, C. 34
Boucher, O. 39
Branger, B. 65
Breastfeeding Medicine 38
British Medical Journal 19
Brown, A. 15, 77, 165
Bryant, M. 111

Cattaneo, A. 43
Centers for Disease Control
    and Prevention 182
Cetin, I. 180
Cohen, R. 112
Cong, Z. 94
Constantine, Z. 45
Coulthard, H. 85
Czosnykowska-Lukacka, M. 42

Dallas, M.E. 78
Davanzo, R. 180
Dee, D.L. 39
Delderfield, R. 24
Dettwyler, K.A. 40, 42, 49, 152, 169
Devenish, G. 65, 66
Dewey, K.G. 40, 113
Doan, T. 94
Duazo, P. 38
Duijts, L. 32

e-lactancia 213
Eglash, A. 115
Elias, M.F. 94

Family Planning Association 162
Finley, D.A. 113
First Steps Nutrition Trust 83
Flower, H. 178, 179, 182, 183
Food Standards Agency 77
Fortune Business Insights 42
Freed, G.L. 16

Garza, C. 216
Gatti, L. 161
Gettler, L.T. 94
Gordon, J. 103, 106, 107, 108
Greer, H. 43
Gunderson, E.P. 34

Hale, T.W. 19, 94
Hamosh, M. 115

Hansen, K. 34
Harris, G. 85
Hassanabadi, M. 177
Havener, K. 104, 227
Henderson, J.M.T. 93
Hesselmar, B. 82
Hicke-Roberts, A. 82
Hookway, L. 95, 165
Horta, B.L. 31, 32

Iacovou, M. 34
Infant Risk Center 183
Information Services Division 112

Jones, L.L. 27
Jones, W. 90, 163

Keinan-Boker, L. 32
Kelly, Y.J. 78
Kendall-Tackett, K. 94
Kent, J.C. 113
Kocevska, D. 93
Kosmala-Anderson, J. 18
Krutsch, K. 19
Kuzawa, C.W. 38

Lewis, J. 165
Lönnerdal, B. 113
López, G. 179
Lorick, G. 211
Lullaby Trust, The 32

Mcfarlane and Ambacher v easyJet Airline Company Limited 118
McKenna, J.J. 94, 95
Madarshahian, F. 177
Mahon-Daly, P. 23
Marquis, G.S. 178
Mason, F. 43
Maternity Action 117, 119
Matsumoto, N. 82
Mohrbacher, N. 149, 157
Molitoris, J. 178
Monasta, L. 180
Moore, M.J. 177
Moscone, S.R. 177
Moynihan, P. 65

Mrtek, M.B. 112
Mrtek, R.G. 112

Nagle, M. 94, 95
Negin, J. 56
Neville, M.C. 113
New Zealand Ministry of Health 38
Newman, J. 165
NHS 38, 115, 158, 213
NSPCC 134

Oddy, W.H. 39
Odom, E.C. 49
Owen, C.G. 33

Pantley, E. 104, 225
Papoutsou, S. 82
Parkin, D.M. 33
Patelarou, E. 33
Peres, K.G. 33
Perkin, M.R. 77
Perrin, M.T. 42
Peters, S.A.E. 33
Pinho-Gomes, A.C. 34
Pisacane, A. 80
Pitman, T. 157
Planned Parenthood 162
Price, A. 93
Public Health Agency of Canada 38
Public Health England 33, 63, 77

Quigley, M.A. 78

Regan, L. 179
Reid, N. 25
Renfrew, M. 29, 32, 77, 78, 112
Rito, A.I. 32
Rollins, N.C. 10, 28, 32

Sacker, A. 78
Sattari, M. 15, 16
Schnell, A. 170
Scientific Advisory Committee on Nutrition 77
Scottish Government 43
Sevilla, A. 34
Shaaban, O.M. 178

Author Index

Shenker, N.S. 40
Silvers, K.M. 33
Statista 43
Steinman, L. 45
Svendby, H.R. 17

Taveras, E.M. 18
Tham, R. 64
Thompson, A.J. 27, 28, 46
Topping, A.E. 27

UNICEF 36, 63
UNICEF UK Baby Friendly Initiative 29, 32, 154

Velez, M. 44
Vestergaard, M. 39
Victora, C.G. 31

Walker, M. 158
Wallace, L.M. 18
Wennergren, G. 82
West, D. 157
Wiessinger, D. 35, 157
World Breastfeeding Trends Initiative 62
World Health Organization 31, 36, 43, 63

Yate, Z. 142